Table of Content

Top 20 Test Taking Tips

1. Carefully follow all the test registration procedures
2. Know the test directions, duration, topics, question types, how many questions
3. Setup a flexible study schedule at least 3-4 weeks before test day
4. Study during the time of day you are most alert, relaxed, and stress free
5. Maximize your learning style; visual learner use visual study aids, auditory learner use auditory study aids
6. Focus on your weakest knowledge base
7. Find a study partner to review with and help clarify questions
8. Practice, practice, practice
9. Get a good night's sleep; don't try to cram the night before the test
10. Eat a well balanced meal
11. Know the exact physical location of the testing site; drive the route to the site prior to test day
12. Bring a set of ear plugs; the testing center could be noisy
13. Wear comfortable, loose fitting, layered clothing to the testing center; prepare for it to be either cold or hot during the test
14. Bring at least 2 current forms of ID to the testing center
15. Arrive to the test early; be prepared to wait and be patient
16. Eliminate the obviously wrong answer choices, then guess the first remaining choice
17. Pace yourself; don't rush, but keep working and move on if you get stuck
18. Maintain a positive attitude even if the test is going poorly
19. Keep your first answer unless you are positive it is wrong
20. Check your work, don't make a careless mistake

General

Medical Terminology

Prefix, root and suffix

Medical terms have three parts:
- Root containing the basic meaning
- Prefix before the root that modifies the meaning
- Suffix after the root that modifies the meaning

Examples:
- Menorrhagia is excessive bleeding during menstruation and at irregular intervals. The prefix is meno, meaning menstruation. The root is metro, meaning uterus. The suffix is rrhagia, meaning a flow that bursts forth.
- Rhinoplasty is a "nose job". The root is rhino, meaning nose. The suffix is plasty, meaning reconstructive surgery.
- Antecubitum is the bend of your arm where the nurse draws blood. The root is cubitum, meaning elbow. The prefix is ante, meaning forward or before.

Whenever you see an unfamiliar term, break it into its root, prefix, and suffix to understand its meaning.

Terminology and abbreviations

There are many reasons on why you must strictly adhere to standardized terminology and abbreviations in a medical office. Following are reasons and where to obtain lists of safe and unsafe abbreviations.
- Standardized terminology and abbreviations are vital for patient safety
- Use abbreviations to save time and space only when there is no potential for confusion over the meaning of your message
- Avoid Latin if there is an accepted English equivalency

Your Medical Records manager decides acceptable terminology and forbidden abbreviations. If you work in a small office and are in charge of Medical Records, use the list of safe terms from The American Society for Testing and Materials' (ASTM) and the list of dangerous abbreviations from the Institute for Safe Medication Practices (ISMP). The Joint Commission on Accreditation of Healthcare Organizations (JCAHO) also has a "Do Not Use" List for medical abbreviations and symbols that are included on the ISMP's more comprehensive list. Post them throughout your office. Use one type of units only. For example, do not use SI units (International System of Measurement) for Lab and Imperial units for Pharmacy without listing equivalencies. Adopt the U.S. Postal Service database's two-letter abbreviations for states.

Medical terminology origin

Most medical terms derive from Greek or Latin, but there are a few English, French and German terms. If you break the Greek or Latin word into its root, prefix and suffix, then you can understand unfamiliar terminology. To avoid awkward pronunciation when there is no vowel between the root word and suffix, add an "o" to the combining form. For instance, add the suffix "metry" (meaning the measure of) to the root word for eye, "opt," to make the word "optometry".

Examples of English terminology include:
- Epstein-Barr virus
- HIV-positive
- 100-ml sample
- oxygen-dependent
- self-image
- English words use a dash instead of a joining vowel

An example of French terminology includes:
- Grand mal (the big sickness) for epileptic seizure

An example of German terminology includes:
- Mittelschmerz (middle pain) for the discomfort of ovulation

French and German do not have convenient combining forms, so you must memorize them.

The following prefixes: ab-, ad-, ante-anti-, be-, bi-, de-, dia-, dis-, en-, syn-, trans-, ultra-, un-

Prefix	Meaning	Example
Ab	from, not here, off the norm	Abnormal
Ad	to, in the direction of	Adduct
Ante	prior to, in front of, previously	Antecedent
Anti	hostile to, against, contradictory	Antisocial
Be	make, aligned with, greatly	Benign
Bi	two, occurring twice	Bicycle
De	away, versus, reduce	Deduct

Dia	transverse, across	Diameter
Dis	contradictory, disparate, away	Disjointed
En	create, put in or on, surround	Engulf
Syn	by means of, together, same	Synthesis
Trans	across, far away, go through	Transvaginal
Ultra	extreme, beyond in space	Ultrasound
Un	opposing, antithetical, not	Uncooperative

The following suffixes: -ficaction/-ation , -gram, -graph, -graphy, -ics, itis, -meter, -metry, -ology/-logy, -phore, -phobia, -scope, -scopy

Suffix	Meaning	Example
-fication/-ation	manner or process	classification
-gram	written down or illustrated	cardiogram
-graph	a machine or instrument that records data	cardiograph
-graphy	the process of recording of data	cardiography
-ics	science or skill of	synthetics
- itis	red, inflamed, swollen	bursitis
-meter	means of measure	thermometer
-metry	action of measuring	telemetry
-ology/-ogy	the study of	biology
-phore	bearer or maker	semaphore
-phobia	intense, irrational fear	arachnophobia
-scope	instrument used for visualizing data	microscope
-scopy	visualize or examine	bronchoscopy

The following four types of abbreviations used in a medical office by health professionals to save time when charting or to be discreet when speaking around a patient; abbreviations take these forms:
- *Brief form* means shortening a common term or difficult to pronounce term, for example:

"telephone" into "phone" and "Papanicolaou smear" into "Pap smear"

- *Acronym* means making word out of a phrase, for example: laser stands for light amplification by stimulated emission of radiation
- *Initialism* means making a word from the first letters of words in a phrase, and pronouncing the series of letters, for example, MRI for magnetic resonance imaging or HIV for human immunodeficiency virus.
- *Eponym* means naming a test or sign for its discoverer, for example, Coomb's test and McBurney's sign

Potentially lethal abbreviations to avoid are:

- *Homonyms* — Same pronunciation but different meaning, such as ileum and ilium
- *Synonyms* — Different words with similar meanings, such as dead and deceased

Reference sources

Reliable reference sources the CMA needs to check correct spelling, selection and use of medical terminology.

- *Abbreviations*: Use safe terms and definitions from The American Society for Testing and Materials' (ASTM). Obtain a list of dangerous abbreviations to be avoided from the Institute for Safe Medication Practices.
- *Style guides*: Provide guidelines for format and presentation in documents. Use the American Medical Association Manual of Style: A Guide for Authors and Editors for an overview.
- *Anatomy and physiology texts*: Contain essential information regarding body structure, function of body parts, disease processes, and common health disorders. Grey's Anatomy is the classic.
- *Specialty texts*: When you need help with specialty transcriptions, try Sloan's Medical Word Book, Tessier's Surgical Word Book, and Pagana's Laboratory and Diagnostic Tests.
- *English dictionary*: Helps with spelling, definitions, and pronunciation. Cambridge Dictionary of American English is the standard.

Greek or Latin medical terms

Most medical laboratory terms derive from Latin and Greek. Most Latinate terms originated from the Greek. The basic rules for pluralizing medical terms are as follows:

Rule	Example
a changes to –ata	Stigma to stigmata Condyloma to condylomata
-on changes to -a	Criterion to criteria Phenomenon to phenomena
-s changes to –des	Iris to irides Arthritis to arthritides
Feminine a ending changes to ae	Ulna to ulnae Concha to conchae
Masculine ending us changes to i	Radius to radii Musculus to musculi
Neuter ending um changes to a	Bacterium to bacteria Treponeum to Treponea
-osis changes to -oses	Diagnosis to diagnoses Anastomosis to anastomoses
-x changes to –ces or –ges	Phalanx to phalanges Varix to varices

Medical and surgical specialties

The suffix -ology means "the study of", and the suffix –iatrics means "medical treatment". Add the body system root to obtain the name of the specialty:

- *Anesthesiology* — Study of pain relief
- *Bariatrics* — Treatment of obesity
- *Cardiology* — Study of the heart
- *Dermatology* — Study of the skin
- *Endocrinology* — Study of the hormone system
- *Gastroenterology* — Study of the digestive system
- *Geriatrics* —Treatment of the elderly
- *Hematology* — Study of the blood
- *Neurology* — Study of the nervous system
- *Obstetrics* — Treatment of pregnant women
- *Pediatrics* — Treatment of children
- *Psychiatry* — Treatment of the mind

- *Radiology* —Study of radiation (for medical imaging)
- *Rheumatology* — Study of rheumatoid diseases, like arthritis
- *Toxicology* — Study of poisons
- *Urology* — Study of the urinary system

Body tissue types

The four major types of body tissue are:
- *Connective tissue* (e.g., bones, tendons and ligaments) joins and protects the organs and keep them in their proper position
- *Muscle tissue* contracts and expands to allow movement and pump blood, lymph, and other fluids
- *Nerve tissue* transmits messages from the brain and spinal cord to all of the peripheral parts of the body
- *Epithelial tissue*, the most common type of tissue, is the skin (integument) covering the body and the lining inside organs and tracts

Body tissue is 55%—78% water, depending on the patient's age and sex. Babies contain the most water. Adult women contain the least. If tissue has too little water, the patient is dehydrated. If tissue is oversaturated with water, the patient is swollen from edema.

Quest. 1

Edema means swelling. The swelling is caused by an accumulation of fluid within the tissues of the body.

- 9 -

Surgical procedures

Appendectomy	Removal of the vermiform appendix
Breast biopsy	Removal of suspicious tissue to detect cancer
cesarean section	Birth through the mother's abdomen
Cholecystectomy	Gall bladder removal
Coronary Artery Bypass Graft	CABG grafts a vessel from the aorta to the coronary artery to relieve angina or blockage
Debridement	Removal of foreign matter and dead or damaged skin from a wound
Free Skin Graft	Detach skin from one body part to repair another
Hemorrhoidectomy	Removal of swollen veins in the anus
Hysterectomy	Removal of the uterus
Inguinal Hernia Repair	Pulling a loop of bowel that protrudes through the groin back into place
Mastectomy	Removal of the breast
Partial Colectomy	Removal of part of the large intestine
Prostatectomy	Removal of the prostate gland
Release of Peritoneal Adhesions	Removal of the peritoneum membrane from abdominal organs to which it is sticking
Tonsillectomy	Removal of lymphatic tissue at the back of the throat

Medical abbreviations and acronyms

Common medical abbreviations and acronyms for these terms you will find in the doctor's notes:

- *AIDS:* acquired immunodeficiency syndrome
- *A.D.:* right ear, auris dextra (* on ISMP's list of error prone abbreviations)
- *A.S.:* left ear, auris sinistra (* on ISMP's list of error prone abbreviations)
- *A.U.:* both ears, auris utraque (* on ISMP's list of error prone abbreviations)
- *O.D.:* right eye, oculus dexter (* on ISMP's list of error prone abbreviations)
- *O.S.:* left eye, oculus sinister (* on ISMP's list of error prone abbreviations)
- *O.U.:* both eyes, oculus uterque (* on ISMP's list of error prone abbreviations)

- *CA:* cancer or carcinoma
  - *CBC and diff:* complete blood count and differential
  - *CHF:* congestive heart failure
  - *TAHBSO:* complete hysterectomy; total abdominal hysterectomy, bilateral salpingo-oophorectomy
  - *CABG:* (pronounced "cabbage") coronary artery bypass graft
  - *DTR:* deep tendon reflexes
  - *D&C:* dilatation and curettage, used to cure uterine bleeding or for early abortion
- *EKG or ECG:* electrocardiogram
- *ELISA:* enzyme-linked immunosorbent assay, used to test for antibodies and antigens
- *fabere:* flexion-abduction-external rotation-extension test, part of a physical to measure the patient's range of motion
- *HPI:* history of present illness
- *Laser:* light amplification by stimulated emission of radiation, a tool to carve tissue
- *P&A:* percussion and auscultation, as in, "The lungs were clear to P&A."
- *PVH:* persistent viral hepatitis
- *PND:* postnasal drainage (can also mean paroxysmal nocturnal dyspnea in a sleep study)
- *simkin:* simulation kinetics analysis
- *p.c.:* after meals
- *a.c.:* before meals

- *h.s.:* bedtime
- *OD:* daily [NOTE: Do not confuse with o.d., right eye.] (* on ISMP's list of error prone abbreviations)
- *ad lib:* freely or whenever desired
- *p.r.n.:* as needed
- *with:* cum or letter c with macron
- *without:* sine or letter s with a flat macron line on top
- *cm:* centimeters
- *cc:* cubic centimeters
- *gtt:* drops
- *g:* grams
- *kg:* kilograms
- *q.4h.:* every four hours
- *mEq:* milliequivalents
- *b.i.d.:* twice a day
- *t.i.d:* three times a day
- *q.i.d.:* four times a day(* on ISMP's list of error prone abbreviations)
- *I.M.:* within the muscle, intramuscular
- *I.V.:* within the vein, intravenous
- *p.o.:* by mouth
- *Rx:* Recipe for the prescription literally means "Take thou". Also called superscription.
- *Sig:* Write on the label for the patient. Also called signature.
- *STAT:* immediately
- *NPO:* Nihil per os (nothing by mouth), a routine precaution before surgery to prevent aspiration of vomitus
- *Auscultation:* Listening to organ sounds to make a diagnosis. Immediate auscultation uses only the ear. Mediate auscultation is with a stethoscope

- *Diagnosis:* When the doctor names or identifies the disease, judging by its signs and symptoms
- *Palpation:* Touching with the hands over the patient's skin to determine the size and consistency of underlying organs to help make the diagnosis, e.g., enlarged lymph glands, hot abdomen
- *Percussion:* Tapping the skin over an organ to determine its condition by the sound it makes

Anatomy and physiology

Anatomical position

The anatomical position is the medical standard used when describing the orientation and location of the parts of the human body.

- A patient in the anatomical position stands with the feet facing to the front
- The hips and shoulders are square and level
- The feet are placed slightly apart
- The arms are held straight at the sides of the body with the palms of the hands facing forward
- The little fingers are therefore nearest the body, and the thumbs point away from the body
- The arms do not touch the trunk, but are held close to it
- The head faces forward, as do the eyes

- 11 -

Four abdominal quadrants

The four abdominal quadrants are:
- Right Upper Quadrant (RUQ)
- Left Upper Quadrant (LUQ)
- Right Lower Quadrant (RLQ)
- Left Lower Quadrant (LLQ)

Six body planes

The six body planes are:
- Transverse plane divides the patient's body into imaginary upper (superior) and lower (inferior or caudal) halves
- Sagittal plane divides the body, or any body part, vertically into right and left sections. The sagittal plane runs parallel to the midline of the body
- Equal halves are the midsagittal plane
- Median plane divides the body into right and left halves. The median plane runs vertically through the midline of the body, or any body structure. The median plane is a type of sagittal plane
- Coronal plane divides the body, or any body structure, into front and back (anterior and posterior sections). The coronal plane runs vertically through the body at right angles to the midline. The coronal plane is also called anterior or frontal plane
- Posterior plane is the back, also called dorsal or ventral

11 body systems

11 body systems and their functions are:
- *Cardiovascular* - Pumps blood throughout the body via the heart and blood vessels
- *Digestive* - Transforms food to energy and eliminates solid waste
- *Endocrine* - Releases hormones into the bloodstream to control metabolism, growth, and reproduction
- *Excretory* - Also called urinary; removes waste products from the blood and expels it from the body
- *Immune* - Defends against all foreign substances
- *Integumentary* - Skin prevents moisture loss, regulates temperature, protects from sunburn, and senses pain, pressure, touch, hot and cold
- *Muscular* - Skeletal muscles move the body; smooth muscle works internal organs; cardiac muscle pumps blood
- *Nervous* - Controls movement, memory, senses, and communicates with the outside world
- *Reproductive* - Allows continuation of the human species and differentiates the sexes
- *Respiratory* - Gas exchange (oxygen intake and carbon dioxide expulsion)
- *Skeletal* - Supports and shapes; protects internal organs; stores minerals; produces blood cells

Digestive system

The main parts of the digestive system in the order of how food passes through them are the following:
- Digestion starts in the mouth with the action of saliva containing amylase to start starch digestion. The mouth also contains the hard and the soft palates
- The 20 primary or 32 permanent teeth are used for mastication of food
- The tongue holds the taste buds and moves the food towards the esophagus
- The pharynx connects the mouth to the esophagus. The epiglottis keeps food from entering the trachea. The pharynx is about 5 inches long
- The esophagus is a 12" tube leading to the stomach. Peristaltic waves start here and moves food into the stomach
- The stomach sac is controlled by the lower esophageal sphincter at the top and the pyloric sphincter at the bottom. Food mixes with hydrochloric acid in the stomach to make chyme. Food normally stays in the stomach for 2-4 hours
- The small intestine contains the duodenum (10"), jejunum (8'), and ileum (12'). The majority of digestion takes place in the duodenum. The small intestine receives bile, produced by the liver and stored in the gall bladder, to digest fats, and amylase and insulin from the pancreas to break down starches and sugars. Digestion in the small intestine can take between 3 and 10 hours
- The large intestine absorbs water and salts, the large intestine consist of the cecum (with vermiform appendix); ascending, transverse, descending, and sigmoid colon, the rectum and anus for defecation. The ileocecal valve prevents food from reentering the small intestine
- Total digestion can take between 24 hours and 3 days

Body parts and their bones

The bones that make up the following body parts:
- *Head:* Cranium made of 8 bones including the frontal (forehead), 2 parietal (back), occipital (back), 2 temporal (side), sphenoid (base of skull), and ethmoid (nasal cavity). There are14 facial bones: mandibular (lower jaw), 2 maxilla (upper jaw), 2 lacrimal (inner side of orbital cavity), 2 nasal conchae, 2 turbinate, vomer), and 2 zygoma (cheek) bones, and 2 palate bones. The ear has 6 bones including malleus (hammer), incus (anvil) and stapes (stirrup) bones in each ear
- *Spine:* 7 cervical (neck), 12 thoracic (upper back), and 5 lumbar (lower back) vertebrae, the sacrum (rump), and coccyx (tail bone)
- *Chest:* Ribs, sternum, scapula (shoulder blade), and clavicle (collar bone)

- 13 -

- *Pelvis:* Ilium (upper), ischium (lower), pubis (front), and 2 coxal (hip)
- *Arms:* Humerus (upper), radius and ulna (forearm), carpals (wrist), metacarpals (hand), phalanges (fingers)
- *Legs:* Femur (thigh), patella (knee), tibia and fibula (calf), tarsals (ankle), metatarsals (front foot), calcaneous (heel), phalanges (toes)

Joints

The types of joints are:
- *Diarthrotic articulations:* Moveable joints with synovial fluid, cartilage cushions, held together by ligaments, like the limbs
- *Synarthrotic articulations:* Immovable joints like the spine and skull

Internal and external respiration

Internal respiration: Exchange of oxygen, carbon dioxide and trace gases at the cellular level.

External respiration: exchange of oxygen, carbon dioxide, and other gases between the lungs and blood, commonly known as breathing.

The passage of gases through the respiratory system is as follows:
- Inspiratory neurons in the respiratory center of the medulla oblongata (brain stem) tell the body to inhale
- Nostrils and mouth warm inhaled air by moving it over nasal conchae and sinuses
- Air passes through the pharynx to the larynx (voice box)
- The epiglottis flips to cover the esophagus
- Air passes into the trachea (windpipe)
- Diaphragm contracts and flattens to raise the ribs as breathing occurs
- Intercostal muscles between the ribs pull the ribs up enabling the chest to expand and air to pull inward
- Trachea splits into the left and right bronchi that connect to the lungs. The bronchi split into fine branches called bronchioles
- Bronchioles end in thin-walled, grape-like alveoli where the red blood cells absorb oxygen (O_2) from the inhaled air and give off carbon dioxide (CO_2)
- Expiratory neurons in the brain stem tell the diaphragm and ribs to relax and exhale carbon dioxide into the atmosphere

Skin

The largest organ of the body is the skin. It forms the integumentary system, along with cutaneous glands, hair, and nails. It has three layers: epidermis, dermis, and hypodermis (subcutaneous or superficial fascia). Its functions are to:
- Excrete salts and nitrogenous wastes
- Metabolize Vitamin D
- Prevent bacteria, parasites, and other invaders from entering the body
- Protect the body from chemicals

- Produce melanin as sunscreen
- Protect the body from water loss
- Regulate body temperature through perspiration, fat storage, and radiating heat from capillaries
- Serve as sensory communication tool through temperature, touch, pain, and pressure receptors

Skin damage

Skin can be damaged by chemicals, impact by sharp or blunt instruments, heat, friction, pressure and radiation. Among the injuries that can happen to the skin are: Abrasions; burns; contusions; crushing; decubitus ulcers (bedsores); gunshot; hematoma; incisions; lacerations; and punctures.

Quest 3

Hyperventalation - a patient breathing more quickly than normal. This rapid rate of ventilation results in carbon dioxide being exhaled at a higher rate than normal.

symptoms that may acompany hyperventalation are related to the metabolic alkalosis that developes. Have the patient sit down and instruct them to take slow, deep breaths.

Patients hands and lips could feel numb and tingly, and the could feel lightheaded - these symptoms are from lack of carbon dioxide in the blood.

Major hormones

The major hormones produced or stored by the adrenals, pituitary, hypothalamus, kidneys, and ovaries and diseases that relates to each gland.

Gland	Hormones	Disease
Adrenal Cortex	Aldosterone Cortisol, androgens	Addison's Disease Cushing's Disease
Adrenal Medulla	Epinephrine Norepinephrine	Anxiety attacks Depression
Anterior Pituitary	Adrenocorticotropic hormone(ACTH) Follicle-stimulating hormone (FSH) Gonadotropic hormones Growth hormone (GH) Luteinizing hormone (LH) Prolactin Thyroid Stimulating Hormone (TSH)	Dwarfism Gigantism
Hypothalamus & Posterior Pituitary	Inhibiting hormones Antidiuretic hormone (ADH), Oxytocin Releasing hormones	Diabetes Insipidus
Kidneys	Calcitriol Erythropoietin	Hypertension
Ovaries	Estrogen Progesterone	Endometriosis Menometrorrhagia

The major hormones produced or stored by the pancreas, parathyroid, pineal, testes, thymus, thyroid, lung, and digestive tract and related disease for each.

Gland	Hormones	Disease
Pancreas	Insulin Glucagon	Diabetes Mellitus
Parathyroid	Parathyroid hormone	Tetany Renal calculi
Pineal	Melatonin	Alzheimer's Disease Jet lag
Testes	Testosterone	Gynecomastia Klinefelter Syndrome
Thymus	Thymic factor (TF) Thymosin Thymic humoral factor(THF) Thymopoietin	DiGeorge Syndrome
Thyroid	Calcitonin Thyroxine (T4) Triiodothyronine (T3)	Cretinism Goiter Myxedema
Digestive tract	Gastrin Cholecystokinin Secretin Ghrelin Motilin	Gastritis Gas-troesophageal reflux

Eye

The main parts of the eye and their functions:
- Aqueous humor is watery fluid that maintains eye pressure
- The bony orbit is the socket protecting the eye
- Cranial nerves that help with the function of the eye such as movement or vision include the optic nerve (cranial nerve II), oculomotor (III), trochlear (IV), trigeminal (V), abducens (VI), and vagus (X) nerves
- Eyelashes and lids protect the eye and sweep out particles
- Extrinsic muscles focus the eye
- The lacrimal glands are tear ducts to moisten the eye
- The lens refracts light
- The optic disc is the blind spot
- The pupil regulates light entry
- The retina has rods for black and white imaging and cones for color imaging, and helps trigger the optic nerve to send impulses to the brain
- The macula is at the retinal center that is very sensitive to light
- The black spot in the center is called the fovea which provides the sharpest vision
- The choroid is a black layer behind the retina that absorbs light and nourishes the retina
- The cornea is the window at the front of the eye that helps with focus
- The iris regulates light entry
- The sclera is tough, white fibrous connective tissue holding nerves and vessels that acts as protection for the eye
- The Suspensory ligament connects the lens to the ciliary muscles of the iris
- The vitreous humor is jelly that maintains the eye's shape and refracts images

Cartilage

Cartilage is a dense connective tissue composed of collagen and/or elastin fibers on the end of bones, which provides a smooth surface for articulation by reducing friction. Hyaline cartilage contains chondrocytes that make it look glassy, and is found in the nose, larynx, trachea, ribs and sternum. Hyaline cartilage makes an embryo's skeleton. Elastic cartilage contains elastin which makes it yellow, and is found in the outer ear (pinna) and epiglottis. Fibrocartilage is composed of strands of fibers that function to help limit movement and prevent bones from rubbing together. Fibrocartilage is found in the knee, the pubic bones in the pelvic region and between the vertebrae in the spine.

Ligament

A ligament is a fibrous band composed of connective tissue stretching from one bone to another in a joint to provide lateral stability. Ligaments also connect cartilages and other structures. Injuries to ligaments are sprains, which are slow to heal and may require physiotherapy and surgery.

Tendon

A tendon is also called a sinew, and connects muscle to bone. Tendons grow into the bone and make mineralized connections with the bone. Tendons transform muscle contraction into joint movement. Tendons can withstand great pressure, but tendons that tear do not heal well, a complete tear requires surgical repair. Damage to a tendon and its muscle in a joint is a strain. Tendonitis is inflammation of the tendon.

Neurons

Neurons are nerve cells that transmit nerve impulses throughout the central and peripheral nervous systems. The basic structure of a neuron includes the cell body, the dendrites, and the axons.

- The cell body, also called the soma, contains the nucleus. The nucleus contains the chromosomes.
- The dendrite of the neuron extends from the cell body and resembles the branches of a tree. The dendrite receives chemical messages from other cells across the synapse, a small gap.
- The axon is a thread-like extension of the cell body, which varies in length, up to 3 feet in the case of spinal nerves. The axon transmits an electro-chemical message along its length to another cell.

Peripheral nervous system (PNS) neurons that deal with muscles are myelinated with fatty Schwann cell insulation to speed up the transmission of messages. Gaps between the Schwann cells that expose the axon are nodes of Ranvier and increase the speed of the transmission of nerve impulses along the axon. Neurons in the PNS that deal with pain are unmyelinated because transmission does not have to be as fast. Some neurons in the central nervous system (CNS) are myelinated by oligodendrocytes. If the myelin in the CNS oligodendrocytes breaks down, the patient develops multiple sclerosis (MS).

Lymphatic system

The lymphatic system is the body's main protection against disease. The lymphatic system is comprised of the spleen, thymus, bone marrow, and a series of transparent tubes that run throughout the body, parallel to the blood vessels. The tubes are lymph vessels, and carry 4 liters of clear lymphatic fluid, or lymph. Lymph circulates throughout the body in the same manner as blood, with valves opening and closing to move the liquid along.

There are about 100 small glands, called lymph nodes, stationed at intervals along the lymphatic vessels. The lymphatic fluid carries invaders to the nodes to be destroyed by lymphocytes, a type of white blood cell. Antibodies are also found in lymphatic fluid. Nodes swell during infections. Plasma from the blood vessels seeps out of the capillaries, immerses body tissues, and then drains off into the lymph vessels. Once in the lymphatic system, the plasma is called lymph. Lymph travels through the lymphatic vessels until it reaches the thoracic duct, the largest lymph vessel, extending from L2 to the neck. The lymph drains from the thoracic duct into the blood circulatory system.

Blood path

The path of blood through the kidney and the path of urine to the outside world:
- Unfiltered blood enters the nephron through the afferent arteriole and flows into the renal corpuscle

- Minerals and some fluid filter out of the blood in the glomerulus, a tuft of blood vessels
- Filtrate enters Bowman's capsule, a shell around the glomerulus, where the majority of filtration takes place.
- Blood leaves the glomerulus through the efferent tubule and enters the peritubular network
- Water and salt get reabsorbed in the proximal convoluted tubule (PCT), and return to the bloodstream
- Filtrate flows into the descending loop of Henle
- Blood continues through the peritubular network and out of the nephron through a venule
- Filtrate flows into the ascending loop of Henle, and into the distal convoluted tubule (DCT) in the cortex.
- Hormones fine tune the filtrate to reabsorb only what amino acids, glucose, and salts the body needs
- Filtrate is now urine, and flows into the collecting duct, where ADH controls its concentration
- Urine passes from the kidney to the ureters, bladder, urethra and meatus for micturition (urination)

Medical terms
- Medial means nearer to the midline of the body. In anatomical position, the little finger is medial to the thumb
- Lateral is the opposite of medial. It refers to structures further away from the body's midline, at the sides. In

- anatomical position, the thumb is lateral to the little finger
- Proximal refers to structures closer to the center of the body. The hip is proximal to the knee
- Distal refers to structures further away from the center of the body. The knee is distal to the hip
- Anterior refers to structures in front
- Posterior refers to structures behind
- Cephalad and cephalic are adverbs meaning towards the head. Cranial is the adjective, meaning of the skull
- Caudad is an adverb meaning towards the tail or posterior. Caudal is the adjective, meaning of the hindquarters
- Superior means above, or closer to the head
- Inferior means below, or closer to the feet
- Superficial is a reference point that refers to an area closer to the surface of the body or to the surface of an organ. A superficial cut is shallow, so it is usually not serious
- Deep is a reference point that refers to an area farther away from the surface of the body, or from the surface of an organ. A deep cut extends through the skin and into the delicate substructure, so it is more serious than a superficial scratch
- External refers to the outside part of a hollow structure
- Internal refers to the inside part of a hollow structure
- Supine position describes the body when it is lying face up or the hand when the palm is turned up
- Prone position describes the body when it is lying face down or the hand when the palm is turned down
- Abduction is a movement away from the midline of the body
- Adduction is a movement towards the midline of the body
- Elevation is the raising of a structure
- Depression is the lowering of a structure
- Flexion is the bending of a joint
- Extension is straightening of a joint
- Protraction is a forward movement along a surface
- Retraction is a backward movement along a surface
- Rotation is a movement medially or laterally around a central axis, as in swinging the arm in a circle
- Circumduction is a circular movement resulting from a combination of flexion, extension, abduction and adduction. When the eyes and limbs move in an arc, they are circumducted
- Opposition is touching together the tips of the fingers and the thumb to grasp an object
- Pronation is positioning the hand so that the palm faces forward, as in the anatomical position. The thumb is lateral in this position while the little finger is medial

- Supination is positioning the hand so that the palm faces backward. The thumb is medial in this position, and the little finger is lateral
- Dorsiflexion involves bending the foot upward from the ankle joint so that the toes point up
- Plantar flexion is bending the foot from the ankle joint so that the toes point down
- Eversion is turning the foot so that the sole of the foot faces outward
- Inversion is turning the foot so that the sole faces inward

Psychology

Piaget's developmental theory

Piaget's theory of child and adolescent cognitive development has four stages:
- *Infancy* — Birth through age 2. The sensorimotor stage, in which humans learn by using their senses, exploring their physical world, and developing object permanence (attachment to the caregivers)
- *Preoperational stage* — Ages 2 to 7. Children develop motor skills, learn to use their imaginations, and develop intuitive thought. They believe in magic
- *Concrete operational stage* — Ages 6 to 11, Children begin to develop logical, though concrete, thinking. Their ideas and expressions are quite

literal because they cannot think abstractly
- *Formal operational stage* — Ages 11 and up. During adolescence, humans develop the ability to think abstractly, with greater perspective, and in multiple frames of reference

Elisabeth Kübler-Ross' theory

Grief is a normal response to the death of a loved one. How a person deals with grief is very personal, and each person grieves differently. Elisabeth Kübler-Ross identified these five stages of grief in her book On Death and Dying:
- *Denial* — This can't be happening
- *Anger* — Why me!
- *Bargaining* — I'll do anything if…
- *Depression* — I just can't handle it
- *Acceptance* — Everything will be all right

Quest. 4

A person may not necessarily follow the stages in order, or go through each stage. A person should go through at least two of the five stages. Patients who have been battling a disease may be willing to accept death to avoid pain, but may not be ready to leave their family and friends for the unknown of death. Family members may disagree on the patient's choice to allow death to occur.

Communication with patients
Expect conflict and tension as your patient struggles with loss. Support the patient and family but do not

impose your personal ideals or beliefs for end-of-life care.

Your patient must first accept the terminal diagnosis, before he or she can retain instructions. When your patient accepts the diagnosis and the initial anger has passed, then your patient is ripe for teaching and treatment.

If your patient is in denial about the diagnosis, he or she may believe spontaneous recovery will occur and may avoid treatment. If denial interferes with booking appointments and giving instructions, ask the doctor to provide your patient with age-appropriate educational material. For adults and older teens, this means outcome data on the appropriate type of end-stage disease. Before every appointment, assess your patient's physical and mental status. Postpone the appointment if your patient is fragile or in extreme pain. Obtain a translator, if necessary.

Defense mechanism

A defense mechanism is a way to cope with anxiety. A defense mechanism protects the conscious mind from intense feelings and thoughts. A sane person uses a defense mechanism to suppress dangerous or inappropriate thoughts from manifesting as conscious actions.

The six types of defense mechanisms are:

- *Rationalization:* The patient justifies an attitude or behavior to make it acceptable or tolerable

- *Denial:* The patient refuses to consciously accept unpleasant realities or feelings
- *Repression:* The patient keeps unpleasant thoughts out of his/her conscious mind
- *Projection:* The patient attributes his own unpleasant thought to another person and refuses to acknowledge it as his own
- *Rejection:* The patient abnormally refuses affection to another person, such as a mother rejecting an infant
- *Reaction:* The patient has a heightened response to unpleasant change, such as nightmares, guilt, mourning, hypervigilance, mood swings, stomachache, or drug abuse

Professionalism

American Association of Medical Assistants

The professional organization that certifies medical assistants is the American Association of Medical Assistants. Candidates must complete an accredited medical assistant training program and write an exam. Topics covered include: Anatomy, physiology, terminology, law, medical records, finance, diagnostics, medication, nutrition and communication. The test consultant for the CMA national certification exam is the National Board of Medical Examiners, which examines physicians. Therefore, employers consider the certification results reliable and valid.

Doctrine of Respondeat Superior

Respondeat Superior is Latin for "*let the master answer*". The Doctrine of Respondeat Superior means if a CMA is involved in a legal action resulting from work, then the doctor is ultimately responsible for the CMA's actions or losses incurred. However, the CMA employee is also held accountable for due diligence. Many doctors prefer to hire certified medical assistants because they trust the National Board of Medical Examiners' input.

Job searching methods

The methods of job searching are:
- Personal contacts
- School career planning and placement offices
- Cold-calling employers
- Classified advertisements
- Internet job sites and message boards
- Professional associations
- Labor unions
- State employment service offices
- U.S. Office of Personnel Management (OPM)
- Community agencies
- Private employment agencies and career consultants
- Internships

Resume and cover letter

The essentials of a good résumé and cover letter are:

- An objective tailored to your target job; correct spelling and grammar
- Relevant skills
- Experience
- Education and training
- Highlights of accomplishments and qualifications
- Truthfulness
- Chronological work history

Interview essentials

The essentials of a good interview are:
- Research; rehearse
- Dress appropriately
- Stay calm
- Counter the interviewer's concerns effectively
- If it is a behavioral interview, answer in a STAR pattern, stating the situation, task, action, and results you achieved

CMA's functions

CMA's functions as a member of the healthcare team, according to the AAMA are:

Clinical
- *Fundamental principles*: Role recognition, aseptic technique, Standard Precautions, sterilization, and quality assurance
- *Diagnostic procedures*: CLIA-waived tests, EKG, PFT, phlebotomy, capillary puncture, specimen collection, and knowledge of radiology
- *Patient care*: Screening, history taking, vital signs, assisting with exams, ensuring

- 23 -

examination room is stocked with appropriate supplies, giving oral and parenteral medications, recording immunization and medication, booking follow-up tests, and emergency response

Administrative
- *Administrative Procedures*: Scheduling, coordinating, and monitoring appointments for inpatients and outpatients; applying 3rd party and managed care guidelines; and managing medical records - Practice Finances: Bookkeeping, billing, coding, and completing clean insurance forms for reimbursement
- *General - Communication*: Adapting for age, disability, and culture; emergency preparedness; patient advocate; network administrator; liaison between patient and physician, knowledge and application of medical terminology - Legal Concepts: Perform within federal, state and local laws, accurate documentation in medical records
- *Instruction*: Patient education; maintain a list of resources
- *Operational Functions*: QA; inventory; maintenance, appropriate computer and technological skills

Communication

Multicultural patients' needs

Respect and tolerate multicultural beliefs and values, even if your patient is non-verbal. Most patients and their families willingly share their beliefs, so do not be embarrassed to ask about their preferences. Ask your supervisor for multicultural sensitivity training.

Obtain a guide from The Association of Multicultural Counseling and Development. Keep a list of translators' phone numbers. Speak slowly while facing the patient and don't address the translator first; be sure to order translations of patient guides and forms. Post pictorial direction signs. Allow multicultural families as much latitude as possible, without causing undue stress for your other patients.

If you anticipate that a ritual will be noisy or alarming for other patients, respectfully guide the family to the Quiet Room. Realize some cultures have beliefs about specific food having healing or soothing qualities. Stay alert for poisoning from traditional Chinese, Indian, Pacific Islander, and Mexican herbal medicines, which often contain mercury.

Americans with Disabilities Act of 1990

The Americans with Disabilities Act of 1990 affects hiring, promotion, pay, and reasonable accommodations; it is enforced at business and service providers with more than 15 workers, on public transit, and with telecommunications.

The U.S. Department of Labor suggests:
- Gain the person's attention before speaking by gently tapping the shoulder or arm
- State clearly who you are. Speak in a normal tone of voice
- Wait until your offer of assistance is accepted. Then listen to or ask for instructions
- Treat adults as adults. Address people who have disabilities by their first names only when extending the same familiarity to all others
- Do not lead the person without first asking; allow the person to hold your arm and control her or his own movements
- Be prepared to repeat what you say, orally or in writing
- Use positive phrases, such as "person with a developmental disability", rather than negative phrases, such as "mentally defective"

Nonverbal communication

Any type of message transmitted between two people that does not involve words is non-verbal communication. 85% to 93% of successful communication depends on nonverbal cues.
- Remember that your patient is likely apprehensive and English may not be his /her first language
- Your patient may have difficulty speaking due to injury, drugs, age, deformity, developmental disability, or the instruments used during a procedure
- Watch your patient's facial expressions, gestures, posture, and position
- Tight posture and/or crossed arms and legs suggest resistance
- Conversely, relaxed posture and uncrossed appendages suggest openness
- Your posture affects your patient
  - Sit closely beside your patient, rather than towering directly over him/her in an intimidating manner
  - Explain what you are going to do
  - A patient feels more comfortable when he/she is well informed beforehand and the CMA works from the side
  - Maintain the proper social distance (territoriality) between yourself and your patient during discussions (about 3 feet apart)

CMA's therapeutic relationship

Your patient shares confidential information with you, which makes the patient vulnerable. At the beginning of a therapeutic relationship, the CMA is responsible for establishing:
- Trust
- Clear, identifiable boundaries
- Mutual expectations
- Confidentiality ground rules

Respond to your patient's needs, but pursue the treatment objectives established by the doctor foremost. Demonstrate acceptance, humor, and compassion to the patient, but keep an appropriate emotional and physical distance. Limit your patient contact to assisting with medical procedures, bookings, and casual conversation. It is unprofessional conduct to date or befriend patients, or give them insider information. Remember: Your primary purpose is therapeutic. Stay alert for:

- Inappropriate emotions imposed on another person (transference and countertransference)
- Conflict of interest (using the relationship for personal gain)
- At the end of your therapeutic relationship, arrange a monitoring schedule, so your patient is not lost to follow-up

Inappropriate communication techniques

10 inappropriate communications techniques to avoid in therapeutic relationships:

- *Ask leading questions* — Never shape the patient's answers to questions, or try to change the patient's interpretation of the situation by "putting words into the patient's mouth"
- *Demand an explanation* — Do not ask "why" questions in an accusing tone
- *Give advice* — The physician advises and the CMA supports
- *Demand an immediate response* — Allow the patient sufficient time for silent reflection before responding

- *Disinterested body language* — Do not appear distracted or make the patient feel inconsequential by impatient motions, bored posture, or rolling your eyes
- *Minimize the patient's feelings* — Do not compare feelings and experiences
- *Negatively empower* — Do not help your patient to manipulate another person
- *Make false promises* — Never promise the patient that the doctor will definitely cure the condition, or make promises that cannot be kept
- *Play into stereotypes* — Racist, sexist, and religious prejudice must not influence your treatment of the patient
- *Deliberately mislead* — Always disclose upcoming treatments, tests, or procedures

Appropriate communication technique

4 appropriate communication techniques to encourage in therapeutic relationships:

- *Use active listening* — Paraphrase and repeat back information transmitted by your patient. Ask for clarification when the message is confusing. Summarize what you agreed to at the end of your conversation
- *Watch for nonverbal cues* — Nonverbal cues are gestures, grimaces, posturing, appearance, and eye movements that comprise 85% of all communication. Nonverbal cues denote pain,

Question 12

fear, lying, depression, or subterfuge by a caregiver. Gently ask your patient to clarify when verbal and nonverbal cues do not match. Children and psychiatric patients may develop tic disorders (involuntary gestures and movements). If you cannot decipher which movements are truly cues and which are tics, ask the doctor

- *Ask open-ended questions* — Get your patient to 'open up', rather than ask questions that require only a yes or no answer
- *Consider influences* — Put communication in the context of your patient's: Developmental age; emotions; values; ethics; health; education; culture; environment; social and family status; and drug levels

Non-therapeutic communication

Seven examples of non-therapeutic communication are:

- *Negative judgments:* "You should stop arguing with the nurses."
- *Devaluing patient's feelings:* "Everyone gets upset at times."
- *Disagreeing directly:* "That can't be true," or "I think you are wrong."
- *Defending against criticism:* "The doctor is not being rude; he's just very busy today."
- *Subject change to avoid dealing with uncomfortable topics*:
  - ○ Patient: "I'm never going to get well."

- ○ CMA: "Your parents will be here in just a few minutes."
- *Inappropriate literal responses, even as a joke, especially if the patient is at all confused or having difficulty expressing ideas:*
  - ○ Patient: "There are bugs crawling under my skin."
  - ○ CMA: "I'll get some buy spray."
- Challenge to establish reality, which often just increases confusion and frustration: "If you were dying, you wouldn't be able to yell and kick!"

Medicolegal guidelines and requirements

HIPAA

HIPAA stands for Health Insurance Portability and Accountability Act of 1996. HIPAA's Title I regulates healthcare accessibility, especially in the cases of job change and loss; Title II regulates patient privacy rights.

Quest. 31

HIPAA requires: *is a Federal act that addresses the privacy of*

- Every patient's medical record must bear a Unique Identifier to prevent misidentification *personal health information.*
- Patients must be given access to their protected health information (medical records) at any time, upon request *Provides details about how personal health inform. must be protected.*
- Only relevant health information can be disclosed to authorized parties
- A record must be kept of every disclosure

- 27 -

- Every patient or the parents/guardian must receive a Notice of Privacy Practices, outlining how the protected health information will be used
- Physical access to protected health information must be limited (including electronic files via password protection or swipe cards, firewall, and SSL encryption)
- Retired electronic equipment must have all data records wiped clean

Incoming telephone calls

The medical assistant answers the telephone within three rings. Identify yourself: "Good morning/afternoon. Dr. Gentle's office, [your name] speaking." Record the caller's name, number, and detailed information in the day log. Do not put a call on hold until you are certain it is not an emergency.

Screen the call to determine if it is emergent, urgent or routine. Do not interrupt the doctor, unless it is emergent or he or she instructs you to do so. If the doctor is occupied, instruct the emergent caller to go to the nearest Emergency Room, phone 911 if the caller is unable to do so.

For routine and urgent calls, say, "The doctor is with a patient. May I give the doctor a message and ask him/her to return your call?" Most doctors allocate one hour per day to return phone calls and prepare prescriptions for the assistant to fax to pharmacies. Do not give medical advice yourself. Ask the routine or urgent caller to

make an appointment. Do not release test results over the phone, unless the doctor instructs you to do so. Pass along urgent messages to the doctor before routine messages.

CMA's medical practice acts

The scope of practice for medical assistants varies by state. Here are the applicable acts for CMAs:
- Arizona
  Arizona Administrative Code: R4-16-4 Medical Assistants
- California
  Medical Board of California: Medical Assistants
- Florida
  2008 Florida Statutes: 458.3485 Medical Assistant
- Illinois
  "Illinois Nurse Law Safeguards Physician Delegation to Medical Assistants"
- Maryland
  Code of Maryland Regulations: 10.32.12
- New Jersey
  New Jersey Board of Medical Examiners: 13:35-6.4
- Ohio
  Ohio Administrative Code: 4731-23 Delegation of Medical Tasks
- South Dakota
  South Dakota Board of Nursing: Medical Assistants
- Virginia
  "Virginia Law Permits Delegation to Unlicensed Professionals"

- If your state is not listed above, contact the Legal Counsel at the AAMA at http://www.aama-ntl.org/employers/ma_do.aspx/

CMA certification

A CMA must follow the Code of Ethics and bylaws published by the Certifying Board of the American Association of Medical Assistants in December 2009 at http://www.aama-ntl.org/resources/library/aama_bylaws.pdf.

The CMA candidate is ineligible if he/she does not complete an accredited course of study and pass the certification exam. If the candidate attempts to obtain certification by making fraudulent or deceptive statements, or by copying answers, or by unauthorized possession of exam materials, then the Board will refuse certification. If the candidate was guilty of a felony, then the Certifying Board will examine the case and decide on an individual basis.

A CMA can have his/her exam invalidated, or can be reprimanded, or can be put on probation, or can lose certification for:
- Possessing, using, prescribing, or selling illegal drugs
- Violating AAMA ethics, policies, procedures or regulations
- Failing to cooperate with a disciplinary investigation
- The following terms:
- Advance directive
- Code Blue
- DNR order

Advance directive

Advance directive is a legal document in which the patient communicates to his/her family and physician what kind of medical intervention he/she desires.
- A living will is a type of advance directive that terminally ill patients often make
- Specific laws regarding advance directives vary by state, but the patient must always be competent

Code blue

Code blue is when the adult patient is in cardiac arrest.
- Call the resuscitation team immediately
- Sometimes called Code 10
- Code Pink refers to infant cardiac arrest

DNR order

DNR order stands for "Do Not Resuscitate", a type of advance directive.
- A DNR order must be written in the patient's chart by the attending physician in order to be valid
- All discussions with the patient and the family should be clearly documented in the chart
- In the absence of a written DNR order, call a full Code Blue and proceed with resuscitation

Anatomical gift

Anatomical gift is The Uniform Anatomical Gift Act of 1968 facilitates organ transplantation under one standard, which is important when organs are transported across state lines. The Act was revised in 1987 and 2006 to cover transplants from cadavers and fetuses only through the national Organ Procurement and Transplantation Network (OPTN). Organ donations from living donors have many ethical and legal pitfalls, and are addressed in separate laws by each state.

Reportable incident

Reportable incident is a dangerous event that must be reported to the supervisor or Safety Officer within a specific time frame, usually 24 hours to 5 days. Reportable incidents include:

- Medication errors
- Failure to assess and treat a patient according to state protocols, especially if it results in serious injury or death
- Injuries or death while in care (e.g., attempted suicide)
- Inappropriate use of a device or drug that results in death or injury
- Motor vehicle accident resulting in death or injury
- Suspicion of drug or alcohol abuse by a healthcare provider
- Acts or omissions that threaten public safety or result in poor patient outcome

ADA

Americans with Disabilities Act (ADA) of 1990:

- Prevents discrimination in employment
- Ensures access to public services, accommodations, and goods
- Provides sophisticated telecommunication services to facilitate the hearing and speech impaired.
- Requires medical offices to have ramps, entryways, and at least one treatment room that provides access and accommodates the needs of the disabled
- Applies to facilities with more than 15 employees, but all medical offices should strive to comply with ADA

CLIA

Clinical Laboratory Improvement Amendment (CLIA) of 1988:

- Private research labs are exempt

CMS

All other laboratories are controlled by the Centers for Medicare and Medicaid (CMS) and must:

- Be certified or licensed by an authorized accrediting body or the state
- Participate in proficiency testing and quality control, including positive and negative controls
- Have written procedures and policies, and requirements for

monitoring, assessing, and correcting pre-and post-analytical problems

- Retain patient samples and records for specified times
- Toxicology tests require a CLIA number for data forwarding
- How OSHA and the FDA affect medical assistants

OSHA

The U.S. Department of Labor's Occupational Safety and Health Administration (OSHA) set standards for:

- Proper hand washing
- Wearing gloves and other personal protective equipment (PPE)
- Bagging specimens in biohazard bags
- Disposing of needles and lancets in a sharps safe
- Cleaning up spills to prevent spread of bloodborne pathogens
- Harmful chemical control
- Safe equipment use
- Adequate work space
- You must check for updates regularly at OSHA's Web site at http://www.osha.gov and are required to adopt them as part of your standards of practice.
- The U.S. Food & Drug Administration (FDA):
- Assigns the official (generic) name for drugs when it approves them
- Reports recalls and adverse events through MedWatch
- Publishes a free, downloadable Orange Book of approved drugs at

http://www.accessdata.fda.gov/scripts/cder/ob/default.cfm
- Divides drugs into five schedules, based on their potential for abuse, numbered Schedule I (illegal) to Schedule V(benign)
- Sets the temperature regulations for dish sanitization

DEA

DEA stands for Drug Enforcement Agency. Medical offices are targeted by drug addicts for syringes and narcotics, so the assistant may need to contact the DEA and local police. Medical assistants must be familiar with government sites that list drugs, so they can stay up-to-date with the industry, and spell and classify drugs correctly:

- US Drug Enforcement Agency Drug Scheduling http://www.usdoj.gov/dea/pubs/scheduling.html
- FDA Electronic Orange Book http://www.fda.gov/cder/ob/default.htm
- FDA National Drug Code Directory http://www.fda.gov/cder/ndc/database/default.htm
- US National Library of Medicine (Medline) http://www.nlm.nih.gov/medlineplus/druginformation.html
- US Pharmacopeia http://www.usp.org/aboutUSP/

- 31 -

IRS

IRS stands for Internal Revenue Service. It is responsible for tax collection and tax law enforcement. Often, the medical assistant is responsible for payroll in a small office, and must be familiar with IRS withholding requirements. The medical assistant can obtain IRS forms from http://www.irs.gov/.

CMA common work injury

Most CMAs perform phlebotomy (blood collection from a vein). About 43% of phlebotomists suffer annual needle stick injuries. There is a 30% chance the phlebotomist will develop Hepatitis B following a needle stick injury; a 10% chance of Hepatitis C, and a 0.3% chance of HIV infection. Rarely does the phlebotomist contract bacterial, viral, or fungal infections, but it is possible. Keep your immunizations up-to-date, particularly for Hepatitis B and tetanus. Follow OSHA bloodborne pathogens standards. If you do have a needle stick injury:
- Let it bleed freely
- Wash the wound immediately with povidone-iodine
- Report it within 24 hours to your employer. You are entitled to a confidential medical evaluation and follow up
- Fill out Workers' Compensation forms and keep copies
- If you are breastfeeding, stop until your doctor advises you otherwise

- Request prophylactic Hepatitis B immune globulin (HBIG) to boost your antibodies. This may help even if your immunization did not include Hepatitis. If you know which patient contacted the particular sharp that cut you, request disclosure of his/her disease status. Your employer is legally obligated to determine whether the source was infected with hepatitis B or HIV if logistically possible. You are also entitled to blood screening as a precaution
- If the patient is HIV+, consider taking AZT and getting antibody tests at baseline, three months, and six months after exposure. There are health and insurance risks associated with this decision, so consult your doctor first

Federal government healthcare insurance programs

The federal government provides healthcare coverage through two major plans: Medicare and Medicaid.
- Medicare is available for: Seniors who are 65 years or older; patients with specific ailments, such as end-stage renal disease (ESRD); and patients receiving disability benefits for a minimum of 24 months
- Medicaid is jointly provided by state and federal governments, and is available to welfare recipients, low-income children under 5, pregnant

women, and other indigent populations

- Per The Balanced Budget Act of 1997, states provide health insurance for children (SCHIP) up to age 19, in families that may not be eligible for Medicaid
- The Department of Defense provides healthcare for active and retired military personnel and their families under the Tricare program, previously CHAMPUS
- Workers' Compensation insurance is provided under laws generated by each state, to cover medical expenses and lost income for workers injured on the job, or to their survivors if the injury results in death

MPI

MPI (Master patient index) is a database associating the patient's name with his/her unique identifier. A unique identifier is assigned for confidentiality, security and filing accuracy. A unique identifier can be a medical record number (MRN), specimen, number, study number, or insurance number.

Registration record

Registration Record: Sufficient demographic information is collected before service is rendered, including name, address, date of birth, next of kin, payment arrangements, and a unique patient identification number.

Consent to treatment

Consent to treatment is required for all treatment, unless the patient is unconscious or an unaccompanied minor in an emergency. Patient agrees to receive basic, routine services, diagnostic procedures, and medical care.

Consent to release information

Consent to release information is when a patient's signature authorizes release of health information between provider and other entities, such as third party payers. Design of this form should be carefully considered, and may include language translation (verbal and/or written).

PA

The supervisor conducts a performance appraisal (PA) with a staff member to:
- Confirm hiring
- Promote
- Schedule training or remediation
- Reward
- Refer to the Employee Assistance program
- Discipline

A Human Resources rep and/or the union shop steward may be present, particularly if discipline may result. The employee's first PA occurs at the end of the probationary period (3 months or 6 months) and annually thereafter. The written appraisal may include a rating scale, checklist, productivity studies, and narrative.

The supervisor must be acquainted with the employee and observe him/her at work. The PA is based on objective data from performance improvement measures. The employee must comply with published standards. The job description should include expectations and goals related to performance. The written PA should indicate compliance with performance expectations. The supervisor discusses the PA results with the employee and allows him/her to respond with new goals, based on findings from performance improvement measures and related to the organization's strategic plans.

Patient charting

Write legibly in black or dark blue ink only. Never use erasable ink or pencil, or inks that do not photocopy well. Do not use correction fluid or erase an entry. If you make an error, strike it through, write the correction above, and initial your change. Write only at the time you deliver care. Backdating, or adding to previous notes, or making entries on behalf of another healthcare provider are considered tampering.

Strive to chart all pertinent information in a factual manner in the medical record. Do not express opinions or make derogatory remarks, as the record is subpoenable to court.

Illegal documentation actions include:
- Charting actions in advance of performing them (the exception to this is documentation of the care/treatment plan)
- Deliberately omitting details regarding the patient's care, reactions to interventions, and other important information
- Falsifying information (signatures, patient updates, medications, interventions, time and date)
- Destroying any part of a patient's record
- Revealing the contents or leaving them accessible to unauthorized persons
- Allowing multiple copies of the same chart

Obtaining patient consent

Informed consent protects patients by ensuring they or those legally responsible for them are fully educated about tests, treatments, and procedures. The patient has the legal right to know about his/her own condition. The exceptions are life-threatening emergencies and legal incompetence.
- Informed consent protects healthcare professionals from battery lawsuits
- Informed consent is obtained when the patient is given written information in regards to the treatment plan, risks, benefits, and alternative treatment options, the provider truthfully answers any questions, and the patient/parent/guardian comprehends the discussion
- The patient or legal guardian then voluntarily signs the consent form, without duress or coercion

- 34 -

- You must obtain signed consent from the parent/guardian before treatment commences
- Moreover, it is advisable to obtain the minor patient's assent prior to the procedure
- Always keep the original informed consent form in the patient's chart
- Assent should also be recorded in the medical record

Health insurance rescission

In June, 2009 Congress held hearings regarding insurance companies' rescission (cancellation) of private health insurance coverage when policyholders developed catastrophic illnesses requiring expensive treatment, claiming patients withheld information about previously existing medical conditions. In many cases, the pre-existing conditions did not have anything to do with the catastrophic illness, and the patients' doctors did not inform them because the pre-existing conditions were inconsequential. Often, coverage for an entire family was rescinded, based on the undisclosed pre-existing condition of one member. Many cases involve breast cancer, leukemia, and HIV.

A landmark case (Mitchell v. Fortis Insurance Company, Opinion No. 26718, 2009 Westlaw 2948558, South Carolina Supreme Ct., September 14, 2009) found a rescission was based on an incorrect date in the patient's chart and awarded damages for bad faith rescission and reprehensible conduct. The medical assistant must consult with the doctor about pursuing the terminally ill patient whose insurance was rescinded. The Obama Administration is considering banning rescission for pre-existing conditions.

Medical jurisprudence

Jurisprudence is the legal system set up and enforced at various governmental levels. Civil and criminal laws that pertain to medical situations are medical jurisprudence. Medical jurisprudence also involves applying the science of medicine to legal issues such as forensics or paternity testing. Civil laws are more often invoked in the medical setting, as they pertain to either contracts or torts.

Contract

A contract is an enforceable covenant between two or more competent individuals. An agreement between a doctor and his or her patient is a contract. It can be an expressed contract, with written or verbal terms, or it can be an implied contract, where actions create the contract.

Tort law

Tort law governs the other branch of civil law. Torts relate to standards of care and wrongful actions that cause injury to a patient.

Criminal laws

Criminal laws speak to crimes that endanger society in general. There are occasions when criminal law may apply to medicine, usually resulting in fines, incarceration, and discipline by the state medical board.

Medical practice situations

There is an expressed or an implied contract between the doctor and patient. The medical assistant and other personnel are the doctor's agents. The doctor is ultimately responsible for breach of contract under the Doctrine of Respondeat Superior. Nevertheless, the assistant's words or actions regarding care are legally binding upon the doctor. Breach of contract is failure to fulfill and complete the terms of the contract. There are four situations where a contract can be legally abandoned:

- The patient releases the doctor by failure to return for treatment; ideally, the patient sends the doctor a certified letter of discharge, but this is not required
- The patient/guardian does not comply with specific instructions from the doctor regarding care
- The patient no longer requires treatment
- The doctor formally withdraws from the case by sending a certified letter to the patient explaining the situation, to preclude any charges of patient abandonment

Patients' rights information

The Advisory Commission on Consumer Protection and Quality on Health Care Industry, an initiative under President Clinton, outlined eight rights and responsibilities of American patients, as follows:

- The right to information
- The right to choose
- The right to access emergency services
- The right to fully participate in decisions regarding one's own health care
- The right to care without discrimination
- The right to privacy
- The right to speedy complaint resolution
- The responsibility for maintaining one's health to retain those rights

The American Hospital Association replaced its Patients' Bill of Rights in April 2008 with a brochure called The Patient Care Partnership, available in many languages. Obtain a free copy for your patient at http://www.aha.org.

Additionally, the Health Insurance Portability and Accountability Act (HIPAA) include provisions for patient's rights. Information can be found at http://www.hhs.gov/ocr/

HMO

HMO stands for Health Maintenance Organization. It is also known as "managed care". An HMO is a collection of doctors, allied healthcare providers, and hospitals that receive fixed monthly payments from the government to care for Medicaid patients or from an employer for its workers, rather than fee-for-service. Cost control is of major importance to the HMO. There are variations of HMOs, called preferred provider organizations (PPO) or point-of-service plans (POS).

Up until the 1980s, most patients had indemnity insurance that was fee-for service. The patient would co-pay for medical care with an insurance company, and had the option of visiting any licensed care provider. Today, more than 50% of Americans deal with HMOs as a cost-saving measure for government, insurers and employers. Care at an HMO costs a fraction of that with traditional providers, but the patient can only see providers and get tests that are "in-network". Patients do not have to pay up front, fill out claim forms, or wait to be reimbursed at an HMO.

Statute of limitations

Statute of limitations is a law defining the maximum period the complainant or appellant can wait before filing a lawsuit. The limitation date varies according to the type of case and if it falls within state or federal jurisdiction. Usually, the limitation is 1 to 6 years. Homicide has no limitation. If the complainant misses the deadline, then the right to sue is "stats barred" (dead). Rarely, a judge will "toll" (extend) the deadline if the injury was discovered late or a trusted person hid misuse of funds or failure to pay. Minors' rights to bring negligence charges are tolled until the age of 18.

Assumption of risk

Assumption of risk:
- A defense against an accusation of negligence. The defendant

states the situation was obviously hazardous, so the complainant should have realized injury could result
- An insurance company takes the risk of extending coverage, realizing the policyholder might make a claim, but it is statistically more likely to make a profit from the premiums

Arbitration agreement

Arbitration agreement is when the patient agrees to give up the right to sue the doctor. An arbiter (arbitrator) awards damages if injury results. Settlement is faster for the patient, and the doctor gets a malpractice insurance discount. Both parties save on legal fees.

Negligence

Negligence is taking an unreasonable, careless action that could cause harm. Failing to exercise due care for others that a prudent, reasonable person would do. Negligence is accidental. Negligence is not an intentional tort, such as trespass or assault. Business errors, miscalculations, and failure to act can be negligent.

Contributory negligence

Contributory negligence is if a person is injured partially because of his/her own negligence — even if it is slight — then the person who caused the accident does not pay any damages (money) to the injured person. Forty-four states recognize that applying the rule of contributory negligence could lead to unfair acquittal of genuinely negligent defendants, so they now use a comparative negligence test as a more balanced approach. In the 6 states that still have contributory negligence rules, juries tend to ignore it as not being fair.

Comparative negligence

Comparative negligence is a rule used in accident cases to calculate the percentage of responsibility of each person (joint tortfeasors) directly involved in the accident. Damages (money compensation) are awarded based on a complex formula.

Terminating patient's care

Regardless of the CMA's personal opinion, it is his or her responsibility as a healthcare professional to support and respect the choices made by the patient and family. If the family's choices conflict with the CMA's strong personal opinions related to care, then the CMA must terminate care, after giving adequate written notice to the patient and physician to avoid charges of patient abandonment. The CMA is legally required to wait until relieved by another member of the healthcare team who has equal or greater training. Examples of common conflicts that arise are:
- Parents refuse blood transfusions, pain relief, and treatments for minors
- Safety hazards (e.g., a dangerous dog, sexual harassment, or threats)

- Patient will not or cannot pay bills because of insurance problems
- Patient is unruly and obnoxious.

Defamation

Defaming a person exposes him or her to public ridicule or tarnishes his or her memory through untrue and malicious statements. The defamed person can lose business due to loss of his or her good name.

Slander

Slander is an oral statement that damages someone's reputation. It is a form of defamation.

Libel

A written statement that harms an individual's character, name, or reputation; a defamatory libel statement may be true, but is published maliciously (without just cause).

Invasion of privacy

Invasion of privacy is an unsolicited or unauthorized exposure of patient information.

Malpractice

Malpractice is professional misconduct, resulting in failure to provide due care. Most malpractice lawsuits are related to professional negligence, the failure to perform what is considered standard care.

Fraud

Fraud is intentional dishonesty for unfair or illegal gain.

Assault and battery

Assault and battery is declaring or threatening your intent to touch a patient inappropriately or to cause physical harm; battery is the actual act of inappropriate touching.

Subpoena duces tecum

Subpoena duces tecum literally means bring [it] with you under penalty of punishment. It is a court order for a witness to produce documents. The judge must carefully consider if subpoena duces tecum transgresses the patient's HIPAA rights.

The physician and other health professionals must report to authorities:
- Gunshot wounds
- Possible terrorist incidents, especially if they involve the spread of disease
- Known or suspected abuse of a child, senior, or disabled person
- Sexual assault of a juvenile or disabled person
- Poisoning
- Wounds intentionally caused by knives and sharp objects
- Criminal violence, including domestic violence
- Client-specific information for the central cancer registry
- Specific contagious diseases determined by each state

The CMA must keep a written record of the patient's information that was disclosed to authorities.

Administrative

Data entry

Rough draft proofreading

To create accurate documents, a medical assistant must be adept at proofreading. The basic steps of proofreading a document are:

- *Read backwards* — Three complete readings of a document are required. During the first reading, look for errors in punctuation and spelling, and word repetition with a software spellchecker. In the second reading, look for layout, grammar and style mistakes and add new words to the custom dictionary in your spellchecker. In the third reading, consider syntax. Ensure the document flows in logical sequence, and is easy to read and understand
- *Correct* — Check questionable words with these references: Medical dictionary; English dictionary; drug compendium; spelling, grammar, and punctuation checking software; thesaurus; and directories (books or on-line) with the current addresses of doctors, hospitals, and clinics with which you deal
- *Revise* — Query the doctor in square or triangular brackets or use Word's comment feature
- *Create an error analysis chart*: Keep a record of mistakes to save time in future

Greek characters for medical dictations

To find Greek characters and mathematical symbols in Microsoft Word, choose Insert > Symbol > More Symbols. Scroll through the Subsets.

To type the equation in Microsoft Word, choose Insert > Equation > and either Built-In or Insert New Equation.

Character	Pronunc-iation	Character	Pronunc-iation
α A	alpha	τ T	tau
β B	beta	υ Y	upsilon
γ Γ	gamma	φ Φ	phi
δ Δ	delta	χ X	chi
ε E	epsilon	ψ Ψ	psi
ζ Z	zeta	ω Ω	omega
η H	eta	θ Θ	theta
ι I	iota	κ K	kappa
λ Λ	lambda	μ M	mu
ν N	nu	ξ Ξ	xi
o O	omicron	π Π	pi
ρ P	rho	σ Σ	sigma

Microsoft Word 2007

Envelopes
To set up for envelopes using first double click on the icon for Microsoft Word 2007.

- Click on the mailings tab then double click on envelopes in the box in the upper left hand corner
- Type in the delivery address in the first box then type in the return address in the second box

- Click on print preview to set up envelope options based on envelope size
- The font for both the delivery address and return address can be adjusted here
- Click on printing properties to determine proper feed method for the envelope based on the type of printer you are using

Memo template

Your Internet connection must be on to download a Microsoft template. Otherwise, you must set up the document from scratch, which is time consuming.

- Start Microsoft Word 2007 by double-clicking on its icon
- Click the Microsoft Office Button in the top left of your screen
- Choose new
- A dialog box appears
- In the Templates scroll box on the left side, scroll to Memos and click it
- Your computer will connect to Microsoft Office Online via the Internet
- Memo templates will appear

Choose a conservative design: To magnify the memo template for closer inspection, click on a thumbnail in the center panel, and it will appear enlarged in the right panel.

- Avoid busy, colorful, or casual designs
- Remember, your document may later be subpoenaed to court and read by a judge and lawyers
- Choose a design that reflects professionalism

- Double-click the design of your choice to download
- Word 2007 automatically fills in today's date and prompts you where to type specific information
- Note that no signature appears on a memo because it is an internal document
- The dictator initials beside his/her name in the heading

Medical transcriptions set-up

Here is the standard set-up for any transcription:

- 8.5" X 11.5" white bond paper with black ink
- Margins at least 1" on all sides
- Portrait orientation
- Headings flush with the left margin, except for manuscripts, in which they are centered
- Double space between heading lines, paragraphs, and below the last line of the message
- Triple space before the memo, report, or chart message
- Most medical offices use full block style
- Double space drafts, with 5 spaces indented at the beginning of each paragraph
- Single space the body of the corrected message when it is ready to print and sign
- If the document is longer than one page, type the recipient's name, page number, date, and RE: Patient's Name at the top of each page.

Every document must contain:
- Date (and time if it is an Operating Room Report)

- Unique patient identifier (e.g., medical record number)
- Patient's name
- Dictator's name and credentials
- Typist's initials at the bottom left margin

SOAP note

If your employer does not supply a template, use the SOAP note format for composing Chart Notes. Do not transcribe in the chronological order in which the doctor dictates, but put the applicable parts of his/her dictation under these headings in this order:

- S: The subjective portion of the report is the chief complaint the patient or guardian makes
- O: The objective portion includes all of the definite findings and observations dictated by the physician or nurse practitioner
- A: The assessment portion of the report is where the physician's reports the diagnosis
- P: The plan section is where the physician prescribes the treatment program

Successful and uncomplicated surgery dictation

Providing surgery progressed well, the OR team transfers accountability for the patient to the Recovery Room team. The surgeon dictates a detailed Operative Report. The patient's physiological functioning returns to normal over 1—3 hours, depending on the type of surgery and anesthesia.

The PA dictates a brief Post Operative Note, which is not as detailed as a Progress Report, and can use abbreviations and point form if your facility allows them. Follow SOAP Note format: Subjective, Objective, Assessment and Plan. Include the following in this order:

- Date and time
- Unique patient identifier (e.g., medical record number)
- Patient's name
- Subjective symptoms (e.g., how patient feels; complaints; pain control; bowel movements; passing flatus; diet; ambulating; wound drainage)
- Objective signs (e.g., vital signs; edema; bowel sounds; chest sounds; incision is clean, dry and intact)
- Assessment (e.g., "This 42-year-old white female was alert and responsive after laparoscopic cholecystectomy. . ."
- Plan (e.g., remove Foley catheter; change from IV to oral pain control; advance to soft diet when flatus occurs; encourage ambulation)

Surgery complications dictation

If the patient experienced complications during surgery or has difficulty recovering from anesthesia, he or she is transferred to the Intensive Care Unit (ICU) for close monitoring.

- Vital signs (temperature, pulse, respirations, blood pressure, and level of consciousness) are checked every 15—30 minutes

- The interval increases as the patient's condition returns to baseline
- The nurse may obtain central venous pressures and fluid balance (tracking all fluids that enter and exit the patient)
- The patient is stabilized before being moved to a Step Down Unit
- The patient may move from Step Down back to ICU or to an in-patient unit, according to his/her condition
- The doctor, PA, or nurse practitioner dictates regular Progress Reports with more details than the Post Op Note
- The Progress Report contains the date, medical record number, patient's name, current level of functioning, amount of progress made, age appropriateness, assessments, plan, and includes the dictator's signature
- Avoid abbreviations
- Write in full sentences

Transcribe dictation recorded for a patient hospitalized 24 hours or more
The intermediate recovery period follows the immediate postoperative period and continues until the patient's hospitalization is complete. The patient has totally recovered from anesthesia and the emphasis shifts to healing, maintaining a nutritious diet, and regaining independence. The case manager arranges therapy with the rehabilitation team and home care with visiting nurses. The doctor dictates a Final Discharge Note for any patient hospitalized longer than 24 hours. Do not use abbreviations in the

Final Discharge *Note:* It is not as detailed as the Discharge Summary. Include this information:
- Date and time
- Principal diagnosis that required hospital admission
- Complications that developed during hospitalization and extended length of stay
- Comorbidities present prior to admission that require follow-up and additional resources (e.g., diabetes)
- Principle procedure related to the diagnosis
- Discharge plan, including available resources for home care or community care
- Signature of attending physician

Final dictation when the patient is discharged
The Discharge Summary is dictated at time of discharge. It contains:
- Admission and discharge dates
- Patient's name and medical record number
- Attending physician's name and contact information
- Chief complaint or reason(s) for admission
- History and physical examination
- Laboratory and x-ray findings
- Principal diagnosis
- Description of treatment
- Additional diagnoses
- Description of surgical procedure
- Disposition instructions given to the patient and/or caregivers, e.g., limit physical activity, medication timing,

- 43 -

dietary restrictions, and follow-up appointment schedule
- Prognosis for recovery
- Attending physician's signature and date

Documents required in the chart by law are:
- History and Physical Examination
- Operative Report
- In-patient Progress Note
- Final Discharge Note
- Discharge Summaries are not required for routine births with a normal baby, including uncomplicated cesarean sections
- If the patient's chart remains incomplete after 30 days, then the doctor's admitting privileges are suspended

Equipment

Office equipment

The CMA operates the following standard office equipment:
- Calculator
- Photocopier
- Computer
- Fax
- Telephone
- Scanner

If you work in a large facility, Engineering welds an identification tag to each piece of equipment. The Certified Healthcare Facilities Manager tracks its whereabouts. Security investigates theft and vandalism. Security controls traffic, access, identification of personnel, and creates an environment that is reassuring to persons with a legitimate reason for being at your facility.

If you work in a small office, the CMA records all serial numbers and photographs each piece of equipment for insurance purposes. The CMA creates a sign-out log to track of borrowed equipment. The CMA asks local police and fire officials to perform a review of office security and fire safety. The CMA reports theft and vandalism to local police.

Work order procedures

The CMA sends a work order to the maintenance department secretary by internal mail, fax, e-mail, or phone.
- The maintenance secretary logs and time stamps the work order
- The secretary alerts the supervisor if there are duplicate requests for the same work, and may phone the CMA to obtain clarification for the maintenance supervisor and to get the cost center number (if applicable)
- The supervisor reviews the work order to prioritize it
- Work orders are not performed on a first-come-first-served basis
- Work orders are prioritized as emergency (something that must be done at once), routine (something that should be done as quickly and efficiently as possible), and backlogged

- 44 -

(something that must wait for parts, replacement, or cannot be done right away for some other reason)

- The supervisor may investigate who can do the work at the lowest cost
- The supervisor signs the work order to authorize the work to begin as requested, and follows up to ensure it was completed

Maintenance and repairs

If you work in a large facility, then the Certified Healthcare Facilities Manager (CHFM) is responsible for equipment in all departments. In a small medical office, the CMA is responsible for ensuring the terms of a warranty or guarantee are fulfilled.

- The CMA deals with vendors and ensures that delivery dates and other specifications of purchase contracts are met
- Careful record keeping lowers the risk of a warranty being voided based on poor maintenance
- File all warranty records

Your large facility may have a computerized maintenance management system (CMMS) that contains illustrations and instructions for use of each piece of equipment.

- Scan the warranty into your facility's CMMS. If you work in a small office, keep a manual tickler file to prompt you to schedule equipment maintenance on time
- The tickler file helps reduce the costs associated with a piece of equipment by ensuring it is

serviced according to the terms of its warranty
- Include the expiration date of the warranty on the CMMS or tickler card

Computer concepts

Hard drive

A magnetic disc that stores computer data, also called a Winchester drive. It is faster and can store more data than a floppy disc, flash drive, or CD-ROM. However, it is not as portable as other storage media because it is bulky and has delicate arms with read/write heads. Modern hard drives hold between 10 gigabytes and 100 gigabytes of data. They can usually find data in 12 milliseconds or less.

Flash drive

A small portable memory card that plugs into the USB port, also called a thumb, pen, jump or key drive. Flash drives contain less memory than a hard drive but are more portable. They fit in a pocket and are durable because they have no moving parts.

Magnetic tape

A strip of plastic with magnetic coating that can store up to several gigabytes of data very cheaply, also called streamers. It takes much longer to find data on tapes than on discs because all the data before the point you need must pass through the reader sequentially. Tapes are only used for long-term archives and back-ups because they are so time-consuming.

CPU

Central processing unit (CPU) known as the 'brains' of a computer system which can calculate and perform logical operations; the CPU holds data being processed, extracts instructions from memory, decodes them, and executes the instructions. The CPU is usually a small, square, microprocessor chip that connects to the motherboard at the CPU socket, via metal pins on its underside. The CPU needs a fan and heat sink to dissipate heat. To upgrade your computer, find out which company made its motherboard. Follow the manufacturer's instructions for replacing the CPU on the motherboard.

CD-ROM

Compact disc read-only memory is an optical data disc that stores 650 megabytes to 1 gigabyte, or the equivalent of 300,000 pages of text. You need a CD-ROM player to read it. A CD-ROM stamped by its vendor cannot have information added to it. Avoid buying medical databases on CD-ROM, as they are soon stale dated. It is better to buy a medical database through an on-line subscription, which updates frequently.

Operating systems and software

Most private medical offices use the Microsoft Windows operating system on networked PCs. Hospitals often use IBM mainframes. Radiologists and surgeons often use Macintosh computers because of their superior imaging capability.

- Until 2000, WordPerfect was the most common transcription software
- Most medical offices currently use Microsoft Office software to process documents, including Word, Outlook, Internet Explorer, Excel, Access, and PowerPoint
- Adobe Acrobat PDFs are the standard
- Common billing software packages are ABLEMed, EMR, Lytec, or Medisoft
- The advantages of prepackaged software are that they are relatively cheap and many healthcare providers are already familiar with them
- However, they are not customizable
- Your facility may hire programmers to write customized, proprietary software
- Web-based scheduling and billing packages, such as Medical Office Online, are much more expensive than prepackaged software

If your clinic cannot afford prepackaged software, download freeware:
- Linux operating system at http://www.linux.org/
- Open Office software compatible with Microsoft Office at http://www.openoffice.org

- Billing software at
  http://www.allofactor.com/ or
  http://www.freehipaa.net/
- PDF writer at
  http://www.cutepdf.com/
- How the CMA, department
  supervisor, and IT Department
  work together to safeguard
  patient data

Medical office computers must comply
with 1996 HIPAA Security Standards
for the Protection of Electronic
Protected Information.
- It is important for the CMA to
  recognize potential fraud and
  abuse
- An unscrupulous user may sell
  a patient's information to a
  journalist or detective, or use it
  to stalk the patient, or alter the
  record to hide wrongdoing
- The CMA safeguards against
  computer viruses and hackers
  with regular antivirus and
  firewall updates

EHR

The supervisor ensures only
authorized personnel access
electronic health records (EHR)
through an audit trail. The supervisor
asks the IT Dept. to restrict access to a
patient's EHR. The computer alerts the
supervisor to a security breach (when
someone attempts unauthorized
access to the patient's EHR). The
supervisor follows Standard ASTM E
2147-01, which lists the specifications
for audit trails in manual and EHR
environments. Investigators will see
who accessed a record, when, where,
and previous versions.

The IT programmer can restore the
previous information through
versioning, so that any tampering or
falsification is not permanent.

Computer work injuries

Ergonomics means designing a work
environment that promotes
comfortable, safe, and injury-free
work.
- Your work area must allow for
  full range of motion, including
  sufficient knee and leg room
- Your work surface should be
  28 inches high, except for
  keyboarding
- The best chair has:
  - Five castors
  - an adjustable seat and back
  - a broad base
  - a foot bar and lumbar
    supports
  - armrests low enough that
    they are not used during
    keyboarding
  - a shallow seat to permit
    leaning backwards
- Sit with your thighs at or just
  above your knees, feet firmly
  planted on the floor, and head
  directly over your shoulders
- Position your monitor with the
  top just below eye level and at
  a slightly backward incline
- Position your keyboard at a
  height that allows for relaxed
  shoulders and flat wrists
- Protect yourself from eyestrain
  with an anti-glare screen and
  by looking away from the
  computer for 10 minutes every
  hour
- Use more lighting for dark
  walls and paper handling than

for light walls and working
with computer monitors
- Buy a mouse pad with a gel
wrist support

Menu

Menu is a list of options which usually
appears in a bar at the top of the
computer screen in an open software
program. A right click in a document
produces a pop-up menu. The CMA
selects an option by moving the cursor
over it and clicking, or by pressing a
key.

Field

In a database, such as Access or Lotus,
a field holds one type of information
only. For example, a field could
contain a date, name, address, price,
billing code, or diagnosis. The date
field would not accept a name, and
vice versa. Many fields grouped
together form a record.

Spreadsheet

A math or accounting program that
shows numbers in columns and rows,
such as Excel.

Network

A system of computers linked together
by phone cables to share information.

Password

Pressing a sequence of keys to prove
your identity and open a protected
file.

Records management

Filing systems

Alphabetic
Indexing files from A to Z, in the same
sequence as the letters of the
alphabet. It is less accurate than
numeric filing.

Numeric/terminal digit
Indexing by numbers, especially the
last unit; it is more accurate than
alphabetical filing.

Subject
Classifying, coding and storing
documents according to their topic,
such as Sales Receipts or Surgical
Inventory.

Tickler
Also called a suspense file. Indexing
files according to upcoming actions or
unconcluded transactions, such as
arranging an annual service check by a
mechanic before the warranty expires.

EDP
Electronic data processing; using a
computer to record, classify arrange,
summarize, and report information.

Cross-reference
A direction to the reader to check
another section for a more complete
explanation or related information.

Master
Master is a computer file that contains
long-term information, such as a
patient database or payroll records.
The master is updated regularly and

workers refer to it as the most reliable source of information.

Color-coded
Placing colored stickers on files to identify them quickly, usually so they can be purged easily; for example, medical files more than 10 years old can be legally purged; if all 10-year-old files have purple stickers, then the purging job can be safely delegated to a junior clerk.

American Hospital Association's record retention

The American Hospital Association recommends keeping files for a minimum of 10 years, or 10 years past majority for a minor.

- Consider federal and state statutes and regulations, your organization's policy, and the amount of storage space you have available before making a decision to purge
- State and federal statutes of limitations determine the maximum of amount of time after an event that a lawsuit can be filed

Collaborate with your Medical Records manager on a retention and destruction schedule. Retain the following patient information permanently:

- Dates of admission, discharge and encounters
- Physician names
- Diagnoses and procedures
- History and physical reports
- Operative and Pathology reports
- Discharge Summaries

AHIMA retention of health information

Type of information	AHIMA Recommended Retention Period
Adult medical record	10 years after the most recent encounter
Birth register	Permanently
Child (minor) medical record	Age of majority + statute of limitations
Death register	Permanently
Diagnostic images & x-rays	5 years
Disease index	10 years
Fetal heart monitor record	10 yrs. after child reaches age of majority
Master patient index	Permanently
Operative index	10 years
Physician index	10 years
Surgical procedures register	Permanently

Facility closes disposal of medical records
In the event the medical facility closes, the CMA must carefully plan and articulate transfer of medical records. If your facility is sold to another healthcare provider, then the records usually go to the new provider. If your employer is retiring and his/her practice will not be assumed by a successor, then you can arrange a storage contract with:

- Another healthcare provider
- The facility's attorney
- An appropriate storage facility

- Scan the records so they remain accessible electronically
- The State Department provides other options for dispensation of records

The CMA is responsible for ensuring that:
- The records are as complete as possible before transfer
- Living patients are kept informed if records are transferred

Type

Features:
- Integrated
- Paper-based
- Primarily kept in reverse chronological order
- Episode of care is defined by date, with the latest information on top

Advantages
- Easy access to current information, and the chronology of patient care is quickly apparent

Disadvantage
Does not allow easy access to particular aspects of patient care, by problem or by practitioner

Some integrated medical records do divide lab reports from Progress Notes, making them more user-friendly

Electronic

Features:
- Computer-based
- Any chart order format can be the default in an electronic record, with other formats available through data manipulation

Advantages
Takes up less storage space; can be parsed (arranged and rearranged) for specific kinds of access

Disadvantages
Software and hardware may become obsolete, so a paper back-up is legally required; expensive equipment and training required; requires stringent security to protect from hackers

Type

Features:
- Source-oriented
- Paper-based
- Organized by practitioner
- Keep information in reverse chronological order in each section, with the latest information on top
- If a record is kept in the same order during and after care, it has "universal" chart order

Advantage
Particular aspects of patient care can be readily accessed, such as lab reports or patient response to medication

Disadvantage
Does not allow easy access to particular patient problems, and the

- 50 -

contributions of each department to a specific problem

POMRs

Problem-oriented medical records
- Paper-based
- Contains four sections: A database of standard checklists; a problem list; an initial plan; and progress notes
- The problems are numbered, and the plans and progress notes are numbered to match the problem

<u>Advantage</u>
Provides holistic patient information by problem

<u>Disadvantage</u>
Difficult to maintain

<u>Type</u>
Features:
- Source-oriented
- Paper-based
- Organized by practitioner
- Keep information in reverse chronological order in each section, with the latest information on top
- If a record is kept in the same order during and after care, it has "universal" chart order

<u>Advantage</u>
Particular aspects of patient care can be readily accessed, such as lab reports or patient response to medication

<u>Disadvantage</u>
Does not allow easy access to particular patient problems, and the

contributions of each department to a specific problem

Disaster recovery procedures

Disaster recovery means how best to salvage medical records, equipment, and insurance papers. Most disasters affecting medical records are water-based, like leaks and floods. Before using machinery to test or treat patients, ensure that a qualified Biomedical Engineer checks it for safety. Most supplies (blankets, gloves, bandages, medications, and needles) are unsalvageable. Arrange for their safe disposal. Prevent disaster by training staff where sprinkler shut-off valves are located and how to close them. Take these post-damage steps:
- For small amounts of paper, simply separate and dry out in a confidential area
- For larger amounts, contact a disaster recovery specialist through the Association of Specialists in Cleaning and Restoration (ASCR). Outside service providers need to know what kinds of paper are involved, such as printer paper or coated paper for electrocardiograms.
- Reduce the chance of mildew by keeping the temperature down and the air as dry as possible
- Develop a reasonable estimate for the amount of time needed for recovery, and plan accordingly

Screening and Processing Mail

Incoming mail types the CMA receives regularly:

Type of Mail	Example Carrier/Client
Routine letters and packages	United States Postal Service
Electronic money transfers	Western Union, chartered banks
Urgent letters and packages	Couriers such as DHL, FedEx, Purolator, UPS; bike messengers
STAT specimens and drugs	Taxi-cab; armored vehicle, (Brinks); Bus Express
Facsimile	Private offices, pharmacies, copy shops, postal outlets, hotels
Mass mailings, such as invoices, monthly bank statements, ads, newsletters, and notices	Letter mail Plus, Ad mail Plus, AT&T
Voice mail	Sprint, Bell, Verizon
Interoffice mail	Mailroom, porters, runners
E-mail	Microsoft Outlook, Yahoo! Mail, Hotmail, iPhone, Gmail

CMA and incoming mail

The modern CMA handles less paper today because e-mail and voice-mail replaced most surface mail. Expedite processing so the doctor can deal with mail efficiently:

- Sign for insured or couriered mail and pay postage due from petty cash
- Sort according to urgency the letters, bills, statements, interoffice, personal, newspapers and periodicals, ads and catalogs, and parcels
- Open all mail except that marked "Personal and Confidential". If the addressee no longer works for your company, it goes to the successor if it is business-related; forward personal mail to the last known home address
- Inspect all business contents. If a date, signature, enclosure, or return address is missing, staple the envelope to the letter and annotate it. Tape torn letters. Discard most ads
- Date and time stamp all mail for legal protection
- Read and annotate each piece of mail, especially if it mentions an appointment date, a report being mailed separately, confirmation of a phone conversation, or requests a decision requiring more information
- Present the doctor's mail to him/her covered in a folder to maintain confidentiality, with the most urgent on top
- Distribute, route, or answer the remaining mail, as required

Five tools the CMA uses to prevent mail from getting delayed or "lost" on another employee's desk are:
- *Expected Mail Record*: If you read in the incoming mail that

a report or other item will arrive separately, then make note of it. When the expected item arrives, retrieve the original correspondence and attach it behind the new mail

- *Annotation*: If there is a discrepancy or problem with the letter, write a note to the addressee in the margin. Examples:
  o The amount on an enclosed check does not match the amount stated in the letter
  o The writer asks for a specific appointment time that conflicts with an existing booking
- *Routing Slip*: If your manager wants everyone in the office to read an item, then attach a slip listing all their names, the reading sequence, and the date by which you need the item returned. Instruct the readers to initial and date the routing slip when they read the item
- *Action Requested Slip*: Give informal directions to the reader, such as, "Please handle this for Marie while she is on vacation"
- *Digest of Incoming Mail*: When your manager is away for more than two days, log mail by date, sender, content, and the action you took, such as forwarding a request for employment verification to Human Resources

Process outgoing mail

Cover outgoing mail at your desk with a folder or satchel to keep the addressee confidential.
Delivery price is determined by:
- Size
- Weight
- Shape
- Urgency
- Destination
- Route (air or surface)
- Insurance
- Signature verification
- Contents
- Price changes frequently, so check the USPS rate calculator at http://www.usps.com

Insufficient postage
If you apply insufficient postage, then the item will be returned to you. If you do not include a return address, then USPS will collect postage due from the recipient. Buy correct stamps and envelopes on-line at https://shop.usps.com.

Over 70 lbs
Send items over 70 lbs. by freight carrier.
- The Department of Transportation (DOT) regulates shipping of diagnostic and biological specimens, infectious substances, and anything shipped on dry ice
- Follow standards set by the International Air Transport Association (IATA) at http://www.iata.org, regardless of the distance you are shipping, or the

transportation method (truck, rail, air, boat)
- You need the IATA Blue Pages to fill out the shipping manifest with the IATA shipping name, class, subsidiary risk and UN codes
- You must have a Class 6.2 DOT sticker, and if the biological is preserved with dry ice, a Class 9 DOT sticker

IATA risk groups

IATA's risk groups are:
- *Risk Group 1*: Unlikely to cause human disease in an individual or community, e.g., stool smear for occult blood mail-in card
- *Risk Group 2*: Can cause disease in an individual, but probably not throughout a community. Prevention and treatment are readily available, e.g., stool for O&P, and genital swab for candida albicans
- *Risk Group 3*: Can cause serious disease for an individual, but probably not a community. Prevention is less readily available or treatment is less effective, e.g., a brain specimen for Creutzfeldt-Jakob (mad cow) disease, or a tube of blood for HIV test
- *Risk Group 4*: Can cause serious disease for both individuals and the community. Prevention and treatment are not available, e.g. tuberculosis, encephalitis.

Biological shipment classifications

Classifications for biological shipments are:
- *Class A:* Contains Risk Group 2 or 3, but probably not 4. Shipment almost certainly contains pathogens. Requires a first or second opinion (confirmatory diagnosis), e.g., diphtheria swab
- *Class B:* Small chance of harboring Risk Group 2 or 3. Specimen almost certainly does not contain pathogens. Routine screening or first diagnosis, e.g., routine Pap smear
- *Class C:* Shipment does not contain any known pathogens, e.g., killed vaccines

Scheduling and monitoring appointments

Appointment Schedules/Types

The following schedule types:
- *Stream:* The standard booking method, where patients are slotted in 15 minute intervals. A patient with a complex procedure takes two or three slots
- *Double booking:* Two patients are booked simultaneously. Staff takes the History, vital signs, weight, height, and any standard tests (e.g., visual acuity, urinalysis, PFT). The physician performs a short exam and prescribes. Long wait times can result

- *Wave:* A booking method for dealing with late arrivals. Schedule three patients simultaneously, at the beginning of each half hour. The doctor sees them in the order of their arrival. If one patient is late, it does not affect the other two. The longest wait is 20 minutes
- *Modified wave:* Book two repeat patients at the top of each hour, and tell all other callers to come in and wait their turns
- *Open booking:* First-come, first-served. A booking method for dealing with no-shows and emergencies. Give the patient an appointment on the same day he/she calls. Used by walk-in clinics
- *Clustering:* All patients of one type only are seen in a clinic to increase efficiency, such as diabetics, pregnant mothers, or arthritics. Also called Categorization

No-shows, cancellations, delays and emergencies

Remind patients the day before an appointment is scheduled.
- If a patient misses an appointment, notify your doctor and the referring doctor
- If missing an appointment could compromise the patient's care (e.g., a suicidal patient), you may be required to follow up
- No-shows and cancellations phoned in less than 24 hour before an appointment may be charged a fine to cover the doctor's lost fees

Always have patients' contact numbers handy in your scheduler.
- If your doctor is delayed, ensure urgent patients are seen by the locum tenens (doctor-on-call)
- Never leave an urgent case unattended
- Rebook routine appointments
- If a routine patient shows up anyway:
  - Apologize, explain the absence (e.g., delivering a baby)
  - Estimate how long the wait will be, suggest rebooking, and offer hospitality if the patient decides to wait

Always consider these calls to be emergencies:
- Chest pain
- High fever
- Earache

Ignoring or delaying emergency calls can result in legal action against you and your doctor.
Leave at least 20 minutes per day open on the schedule to handle emergent patients.

Resource information & community services

Requisition to refer a patient for outside services:
- After the doctor finishes the consultation with your patient,

review the written Physician's Orders in the chart before the patient leaves your office

- You may be required to book an appointment with a specialist, such as a dietitian, physiotherapist, or psychiatrist
- You may be required to arrange outside tests, such as audiology, bloodwork, ultrasound or allergy screening
- Phone the outside service to book an appointment on the patient's behalf
- Remember that a debilitated patient is unable to bear more than one invasive test per day
- Obtain the correct requisitions for the tests from the outside services
- Fill them out by accurately transcribing information from the patient's chart to the requisition
- You will find prescribed drugs on the Nursing History Chart
- Send the requisition with the patient to the appointment caution the patient that most hospital Operating Rooms are booked several months in advance
- The doctor may also dictate a referral letter to the specialist, which you type later, and send by fax or surface mail so that it arrives well before the appointment.

CMA's role as patient advocate

A patient advocate speaks on the patient's behalf to obtain services and information, and protect rights. If your institution works on the case management system, it will appoint an advocate for each patient, who is usually an RN or Social Worker. The CMA often spends more time with the patient than the case manager therefore; the patient will sometimes feel more comfortable with the CMA because of this.

Relate the hopes, wishes, fears and concerns of the patient to the healthcare team. Do not become embroiled in emotional family dynamics by revealing confidences. However, expressing the patient's desires through the healthcare team is an appropriate avenue to ensure the patient's voice is heard. The American Hospital Association replaced its Patients' Bill of Rights in April 2008 with a brochure called The Patient Care Partnership, available in many languages. Obtain a free copy for your patient at http://www.aha.org

Look back

"Look back" is record checking, often on microfilm or microfiche, to find old contacts and disease vectors. For example, when your patient tests positive for HIV, the doctor is responsible for notifying Public Health, which then checks blood transfusion records to find out if your patient was a blood donor. If your patient did donate blood, Public Health attempts to find the recipients. Many years can elapse between donation and HIV diagnosis. You may be required to "look back" through the patient's chart for clues to help Public Health.

To make the chart useful for "look back", you need to document:

- A copy of all lab requisitions and test results, including the date and time
- Any no-shows
- Name and contact information of translators used to explain tests, if any
- Signed and witnessed consent forms
- Copies of any patient preparation or aftercare instructions
- Adverse reactions
- Patient refusal of tests and person in authority you notified
- When and to whom you reported the results

Maintaining office environment

OSHA requires that medical offices use good aseptic technique to reduce the spread of disease. Disinfection means cleaning objects to eliminate most pathogenic (disease-causing) microorganisms, such as bacteria, viruses, molds, and parasites. Disinfection and sanitization (washing) do not eliminate spores, which are dormant (sleeping) bacteria waiting for more hospitable growing conditions, or the seeds of algae, fungi, plants, and a few protozoans. The only way to kills spores is by autoclave oven. Autoclaving is appropriate for small instruments but not furniture or other large surfaces.

Prepare a fresh solution of germicidal detergent daily.

- Use the detergent to wipe down soiled walls, mattress covers, furniture, and any equipment that is not the responsibility of Central Sterile Supply (CSS)
- Mop the floors or wet-vacuum them if you do not have a Housekeeping service
- Post the appropriate signs outside isolation rooms
- Keep the necessary isolation equipment outside of the isolation room for staff and visitors to don and doff
- Keep a pump bottle of 70% to 80% alcohol cleanser at the entrance to each exam room and at the front desk

Medical inventory

Your doctor and specialists inform you which medical supply companies they purchase from routinely. Produce a list of required supplies, including:

- Item name
- Size, color, number, units, and cost
- Supplier's name, address, and phone and fax numbers
- The list tells you how long an item lasts, when to reorder, and cost comparisons
- Prescription pads and drug samples are available free from drug company sales reps

Check the drug and supply cupboards against your supply list daily and weekly. Ensure you always have adequate supplies available, but

- 57 -

remember that reagents and drugs expire.

- Reorder before supplies are exhausted from the authorized suppliers only
- Do not order large quantities without the doctor's authorization, as they may stale-date
- Include the price quote on the purchase order (PO)
- Keep a copy of your PO in a pending file until the supplies arrive, for comparison to the packing slip

Always lock the supply and drug cupboards.

- Drug addicts target painkillers, sleeping pills, tranquilizers, and syringes, so consult Pharmacy and Security about safe storage
- Do not flush expired drugs down the toilet because they cause environmental harm
- Call the hospital pharmacy or your drug rep to have the expired drugs incinerated

Tickler file manages equipment

File the manufacturer's recommendations for a preventative maintenance schedule when you buy a new piece of equipment, and put the suggested date in your tickler file as a reminder. If there is no instruction guide provided when you purchase a second hand machine, ask the vendor to provide one, or ask a Biomedical Engineer to write a manual as a resource for less skilled workers.

Start a maintenance log for each new machine purchased, and keep it for the life of the machine or until its tax depreciation is finished, whichever comes later.

- Update the log with a description of each maintenance item performed
- The name of the maintenance worker
- The date and duration of maintenance, along with possible problems and feedback from the maintenance worker
- Keep the log readily available with any relevant publications, such as service and operation manuals, and specialized tools for workers' use
- Inspection and repair records, inspection schedules, and "*as-built*" drawings are also among the resources that should be available

Office policies & procedures

P&P manual

Policy and procedures manual, a binder or company Intranet posting of rules staff must follow, whereas a guideline is an expert suggestion. By law, P&Ps must be readily available to all staff, and your employer must train staff fully to use them. An example is an infection control policy and procedure to control the spread of disease through hand washing.

Algorithm

Algorithm is a flowchart containing treatment pathways for specific patient populations and disorders. The instructions follow an "if X condition occurs, then give Y drug and perform Z procedure" pattern. An expert committee (usually the chief pharmacist, medical director, and nursing executive) authorizes algorithms for posting in the Policies & Procedures manual. Following an algorithm ensures you legally comply with the standard of care at your facility and your patients' outcomes are statistically likely to be better.

Personnel manual

An employee handbook describing benefits, compensation, complaint resolution, discipline, dress code, emergency preparedness, and Human Resources policies that apply to all employees.

Patient information booklet

People who are ill may not retain oral information due to stress. A booklet that answers common questions about a disease or procedure reinforces the doctor's verbal explanation.

Practice finances

Bookkeeping performed by the CMA:
- Petty cash
- Single-entry bookkeeping
- Bank deposits, checking, and reconciliations
- Patient accounts and statements
- Payroll

The CMA completes the financial records when the office is not busy because the doctor is not examining patients. Usually, a Chartered Accountant (CA) sets up the doctor's accounting records and tells the CMA the column headings to use for the cash disbursements journal. The CMA records the:
- Date of purchase
- Reason for payment in the Explanation column
- Check number used to pay for the purchase; and amount
- The CMA usually prepares bank deposits daily, payroll weekly, and reviews the practice finances monthly

The Chartered Accountant also calculates the annual income tax and completes the financial statements through double-entry bookkeeping. Rarely is the CMA responsible for practice taxes and financial statements. Standard coding systems:
- ICD-10-CM
- SNO-MED
- CPT

The most commonly used coding systems are:
- The International Classification of Diseases, Tenth Edition, Clinical Modification, or ICD-10-CM
- Systematized Nomenclature of Human and Veterinary Medicine (SNOMED-CT) by the

College of American Pathologists
- Current Procedural Terminology (CPT)

Some coding systems are classification systems, and some are nomenclatures. Most healthcare organization uses multiple coding systems.
- SNOMED-CT is the nomenclature system with the most potential to handle the complex data represented in electronic health records (EHRs)
- SNOMED offers comprehensive international clinical reference terminology, used worldwide
- The CT suffix stands for core technology
- There is also an older version, with RT as a suffix for reference terminology
- Designed for computers, SNOMED-CT offers a consistent language for capturing, sharing, and aggregating health data across specialties and sites of care
- SNOMED links synonyms to a single concept
- For instance, SNOMED recognizes appendicitis as an inflammatory and GI disease
- SNOMED includes domain-specific vocabularies, such as those for Nursing
- SNOMED maps to interface with other clinical terminologies, such as ICD-9, ICD-10, and others

Medicare part A

Medicare A is no-cost hospital insurance for: Social Security recipients over 65 years old; Patients receiving disability benefits for a minimum of 24 months; Patients with renal failure (dialysis patients) in these facilities: critical access hospitals; home care; in-patient hospitals; hospices; and skilled nursing facilities

Medicare A is financed primarily through payroll tax, and is unavailable to beneficiaries who are ineligible for federal retirement benefits.

Medicare part B

Medicare B insurance covers out-patient treatment for starting at $96.40 per month in 2010 for:
- Blood transfusion
- Diagnostic tests like glaucoma, Pap smears, mammograms, and prostate exams
- Doctors' office visits
- Durable assistive devices, like beds, oxygen, walkers, and wheelchairs
- Laboratory tests
- One physical exam in the first 6 months
- Outpatient clinics for mental health, occupational therapy, and physiotherapy
- Outpatient surgery
- Vaccines, like Hepatitis B and Pneumococcus

- Part B is financed by federal appropriations with monthly premiums paid by the beneficiary, who also pays some deductibles and copayments

Medicare part C

Medicare Part C is also known as Medicare Advantage. It is available to beneficiaries enrolled in Parts A and B (hospital and outpatient insurance coverage). Part C offers various managed-care plans, including HMO, POS, and PPO plans.

Medicare part D

Medicare Part D is a recently added option that provides prescription drug coverage. There are several plans available, but the beneficiary always pays a monthly premium and part of the drug cost.

Medicare providers are reimbursed through an insurance company contracted by the federal government as a fiscal intermediary.

TERFA

Congress passed the Tax Equity and Fiscal Responsibility Act (TERFA) in 1983 to combat spiraling medical costs.
- TERFA created the Prospective Payment System (PPS), a method whereby reimbursement amounts are predetermined based on the services rendered
- CMS annually reviews standardized rates,

represented by classifications called Diagnosis-related Groups (DRGs) for inpatient care, and Resource-based Relative Value Scale (RSBRVS) for physician services

Medicaid

Medicaid is the program through which the federal and state governments help low-income individuals by paying for those medical services that are deemed to be absolutely necessary. Medicaid is covered by Social Security Act Title XIX. Medicaid is available to welfare recipients, low-income children under 5, pregnant women, and other indigent populations.

Tricare

The Department of Defense provides healthcare for active and retired military personnel and their families through the Tricare program, previously CHAMPUS.

CHAMPVA

Civilian Health and Medical Program of the Department of Veterans Affairs (CHAMPVA) is always the secondary payer, after Medicare, to minimize out-of-pocket expenses. CHAMPVA covers the families of vets who were killed or permanently disabled in the line of duty, who are ineligible for Tricare.

Workers' Compensation

Insurance provided under laws generated by each state, to cover medical expenses and lost income for workers injured on the job, or to their survivors if the injury results in death.

Third-party payer

Third-Party Payers are insurance companies or employers that use patient care data as the basis for claims processing to pay for healthcare services provided. Many third-party payers encourage the use of Ambulatory Care by providing financial incentives. It is very time-consuming for the physician to qualify a claim for third-party reimbursement because he/she must specify diagnoses and provide exact details, e.g., a surgical procedure must document the reason for surgery, lesion length, layers of fascia involved, etc.

The CMA reduces the time the physician spends on documentation by reviewing the patient's record the day before an appointment, to isolate the pertinent information. The patient must authorize disclosure of his/her information to third-party recipients. The third-party payer will probably redisclose your patient's information to the Medical Information Bureau (MIB), which allows access to other potential insurers for up to 7 years. Only drug or alcohol abuse cases are exempt. Third-party payers require a Progress Note for each visit billed.

Practice finances

Payer contracts are legally binding documents describing the obligations of both providers and payers. Healthcare billing adheres to industry standards of language and service codes, as noted by the Common Procedure Coding System (HCPCS) of the Healthcare Financing Administration (HCFA).

- A provider who contracts with a payer is considered a participating provider
- If no contract exists, then the provider is considered a non-participating provider, who may be reimbursed less by a third-party payer
- Non-participating providers usually obtain additional co-payment from the patient
- This is especially true of mental healthcare providers, like counselors and psychologists

The CMA deals with occasional third-party payers through surface mail, and with regular third-party payers through a virtual private network (VPN), or Extranet. One component of the VPN is a demilitarized zone (DMZ), which sits between the internal network and the VPN. It allows outside access to a third-party portion of the network, while protecting the Intranet, or internal, information.

Doctor enrollment

Providers must produce specific documentation to payers to obtain billing privileges, for example:

- A doctor must meet credentialing standards established by the National Committee for Quality Assurance (NCQA)

- Individual healthcare providers and business owners must supply the payer with a tax identification number for the IRS

Master charge list

Master charge lists delineate how much can be charged for each service, as identified by a CPT-4 code. These lists are also known as charge master, charge description master (CDM), or fee schedule.

- Charges are impacted by clinical modifiers, which affect reimbursement
- Modifiers are given numeric or alphabetical codes
- Either the CMA or the HIM manager is responsible for monitoring the accurate and timely coding of all services rendered, and regularly analyzing contracted reimbursement rates and expenses associated with services or product costing

Quest. 28

Process a third-party claim – companies that are used by insurance companies to process claims or payments.

The CMA ensures the bill to the third-party payer is complete and accurate, with correct subscriber, patient *The physician may submit a* information and medical codes. The *claim to* CMA generates primary and *insurance company* secondary billing for patients covered *and the insurance* by multiple insurance plans. *company passes the claim onto another*

- The payer rejects incomplete *insurance* or inaccurate claims, and the *company* *that* CMA must submit an inquiry *specializes* and appeal the decision *in processing*
- If a third-party declines *that type of* payment after an appeal, the *claim.* CMA informs the patient that

he/she must self-pay (also called direct pay or out-of-pocket payment)

If you do not receive payment within the time indicated in the contract, initiate a trace.

- Insurance payments are accompanied by either a remittance advice (RA) or explanation of benefits (EOB), indicating the: Billed amount; allowable amount by insurance coverage; payment amount; patient liability; amount disallowed by insurance.
- Reconcile the accounts to ensure the correct payment was made according to the individual payer's contract, which may be based on a percentage, per unit, DRG rate, or other fee schedule

Relative value studies

A relative value study is a schedule that assigns a unit value to a medical procedure to compare costs.

RSBRVS

Resource-based Relative Value Scale (RSBRVS) is the Center for Medicare and Medicaid (CMS) reviews its standardized rates every year. Resource-based Relative Value Scale (RBRVS) are standardized rates the CMS pays providers for physician services.

DRGs

Diagnosis Related Groups is the Center for Medicare and Medicaid

(CMS) reviews its standardized rates every year. Diagnosis-related Groups (DRGs) are standardized rates the CMS pays for inpatient care based on principle diagnosis, procedures, age, gender and other complicating issues.

Contracted fees

Contracted fees is a benefit plan that prohibits extra billing. The participating provider agrees to accept a list of specific fees from the payer. A fee is the total the provider can charge.

Accounts receivable

Accounts receivables (A/R) is money owed to the practice by a patient for services and products the provider sold on credit and for which the patient has been invoiced. Enter A/R as a current asset on the balance sheet.

Billing cycle

Billing cycle is the period between billing for services and products, which is usually one month in most practices.

Aging of accounts

Aging of accounts is classifying the accounts according to risk by the number of days that have elapsed since the due date or billing date. Most practices have an aging schedule of 1 to 30 days, 31 to 60 days, 61 to 90 days, and more than 90 days. The longer an account is unpaid, the greater the risk that the patient will default.

Collections

Collections is the CMA transfers a delinquent account more than 90 days overdue to the Collection Department or a private collection agency. It is cheaper for the CMA to negotiate with the patient than it is to accept 10% of recovered money from the collection agency or risk that no money will be recovered if the patient files for bankruptcy.

Itemization

The CMA prepares a bill for the payer with a detailed list of all procedures performed and products used during one visit for a particular patient. The supplier prepares a bill for the practice listing all products sold in detail (size, shape, quantity, color, material, etc.).

Consumer protection act

A legal statute that prohibits deceptive marketing, encourages the seller to give the consumer information, and enforces product safety standards.

A/P

Accounts payable (A/P) is unpaid bills the practice owes to suppliers. A/P does not include payroll, rent, taxes, or accrued interest. Enter A/P as current liabilities (short-term) on the balance sheet.

Ordering

Ordering is when the CMA issues a Purchase Order (P.O.) number to the supplier to confirm a request for goods or services. When the CMA accepts receipt of the goods or services, the P.O. becomes a binding legal agreement for the practice to pay the supplier.

Invoice

Invoice is a bill of sale or contract that identifies the practice and patient, or the seller and buyer. List the quantity of products or services sold and describe them. Show the date of service or shipment, delivery or transport mode, price, and payment terms, including discounts. When the CMA or doctor signs the invoice, it becomes a demand for payment. When the patient pays the invoice in full, it becomes a document of title.

Tracking

Tracking is monitoring performance or delivery. As a person or product passes through checkpoints, the CMA finds if there is deviation from a benchmark through tracking software.

Bank deposit

Bank deposit is the CMA deposits the takings for the practice at least once per week at a banking institution in one of these types of accounts:
- Current, checking, savings, money market, or time deposit account
- The bank is liable to give the depositor (the practice) cash, less the transaction fees

Clinical

Principles of infection control

Medical asepsis procedures

Medical asepsis means controlling the spread of hospital-acquired (nosocomial) disease and cross-infections (different pathogens passed between two patients):

- Wash your hands for 20-30 seconds using warm water and soap, taking care to clean your fingernails thoroughly whenever visibly soiled, before and after any contact with patients, and after gloves are removed
- Disinfect patient care materials before use with the proper chemical agent, according to the manufacturer's specifications
- Maintain a clean patient care environment, with adequate space, ventilation, sunlight, and cool temperature
- Dispose of infectious material as soon as soiling is discovered in the proper bin (concurrent cleaning)
- Disinfect patient care materials after a patient leaves the office, or dies, or is transferred to another floor or facility (terminal cleaning)
- Use Clean and Dirty Utility Rooms to separate unused equipment from used equipment and prevent contamination
- Store clean linen separate from used linen and limit access to the Clean Linen Room to authorized personnel only

Surgical asepsis procedure

Surgical asepsis means sterilizing instruments, sutures, drapes, sponges, and other equipment used for surgery and storing them safely, so they do not become reinfected.

- Surgical equipment pierces the skin or mucous membranes, or is placed inside a wound, or is inserted into a body cavity that is normally sterile
- Sterility is not required for instruments introduced into the vagina, ear canal, or mouth; a vaginal speculum, otoscope, or tongue depressor can be clean (disinfected), rather than sterile
- Surgical equipment must be free of all microorganisms, including spores

Clean the field where you will sterilize the instruments.

- Wash your hands thoroughly for 2-5 minutes using an antimicrobial soap then glove
- Use sterile supplies only
- After you sterilize the instruments in an autoclave pack, create a sterile field
- Find a clean, flat, dry surface that is free from drafts
- Wash your hands and don sterile gloves
- Cover the field with a sterile drape
- Open the autoclave pack on the drape

- Keep sterile all articles that touch the sterile field

Biohazardous material disposal

Wear a gown, gloves, and mask when handling all tissue.
- Post biohazard signs on walls and containers
- Properly label all containers
- Ventilate Biohazardous areas very well; consult your Safety Officer regarding fume hoods and filters
- Avoid using aerosols, especially for quick freezing tissue, because they increase your risk of exposure to infectious material
- Dispose of all soft waste material in red or yellow biohazard bags, and disposable blades in red or yellow sharps containers
- Disinfect non-disposable objects, such as tables
- The CDC and EPA recommend steam sterilization and incineration for all waste except pathological waste, which only needs incineration
- Dispose of blood in the sink with adequately running water
- If you or a co-worker is exposed to hazardous materials, start decontamination procedures immediately
- Check the written procedures in your policy and procedures manual (P&P)
- By law, P&Ps must be readily available to all staff, and your employer must train staff fully to use them

Asepsis, antisepsis, isolation, and standard (universal) precautions

Asepsis prevents infection during surgical procedures by reducing pathogens.
- It requires sterile instruments and sterile gloves, and a strong disinfectant that can kill both Gram-positive and Gram-negative bacteria and their resistant spores, like 70% povidone-iodine
- Antisepsis is reducing the flora and transient microorganisms on the skin for minor procedures like venipuncture
- Clean gloves are worn
- It requires a short-acting antiseptic like 70% isopropyl alcohol that can denature proteins
- Strict isolation segregates infectious patients to one room, and visitors are restricted
- Modified isolation attempts to limit infection with protective techniques, like donning gloves, gowns, and masks when handling the patient's body fluids
- Reverse isolation protects a patient from others in a clean room, as after kidney transplant
- Standard or universal precautions mean healthcare workers control the spread of disease by assuming every patient's samples are infectious, and following the U.S.

- Occupational Safety and Health Administration (OSHA) standards for proper hand washing, wearing gloves and other personal protective equipment , bagging specimens in biohazard bags, and disposing of needles and lancets in a sharps safe

Correct hand-washing technique

Procedures for hand washing:
- To wash your hands correctly, first remove your jewelry
- Use clean, dry paper towels to turn on the taps
- Use warm water to avoid skin damage
- Wet your hands and apply disinfectant soap (poviodine scrub or bar soap rinsed and stored in a drainer)
- Count to 30 while scrubbing the backs and palms of your hands with the lather, and interlace your fingers while rubbing them together
- Brush gently under your nails
- Note any cuts, rashes, broken or long nails that need treatment before resuming work
- Rinse well and dry your hands with paper towels, not a blow dryer
- Use clean paper towel to turn off the taps and to open the exit door
- If there is no sink nearby, use 70% to 80% alcohol cleanser (Cutan, Florafree, Manorapid, Purell) for 15 seconds, followed by disposable

antiseptic towelettes (benzalkonium chloride)
- Change gloves frequently by turning them inside out from the wrists
- Wash your hands as soon as possible

Treatment area

Autoclave tray preparation

An autoclave oven sterilizes instruments.
- The CMA cleans instruments promptly after use by immersion in an ultrasonic bath or instrument washer
- Instruments that cannot be cleaned immediately are presoaked in disinfectant temporarily
- Use a scrub brush for stubborn debris
- Separate the blades of all instruments
- Ultrasonic solution should cover all the instrument parts
- Instruments that have hinges (e.g., scissors and forceps) should be sanitized first and later sterilized in the open position
- Remove instruments from the ultrasonic bath, hold them under running water, dry, and then wrap them for the autoclave
- Seal the pack with pressure-sensitive striped tape, which turns color when the correct temperature has been reached

- 68 -

- Sets the autoclave thermostat to:
  - Dry heat at 170°C (340°F) for 1 hour for powders and swabs that deteriorate when wet
  - Steam at 121°C (250°F) and 15 lbs of pressure for 30 minutes for most metal and glass

Dry the instruments well prior to storage. If the doctor requests an instrument that is not on the autoclaved tray you prepared, then use a flash prevacuum sterilizer at 134°C (275°F) for 4 minutes to sterilize the instrument.

Electrocardiograph records and EKGs

An electrocardiograph machine records the heart's electrical activity on an electrocardiogram (EKG or ECG).
- The EKG monitors heart rate, patterns of heartbeats, the size and location of the chambers of the heart, and helps to diagnose heart conditions
- The EKG is a non-invasive, painless, inexpensive way to determine if there is any damage to the heart muscle (myocardium) or electrical conduction system
- The cardiologist uses the EKG to determine if drug therapy or pacemaker implants are having the desired effect
- The P wave on an EKG corresponds to the atria contracting

- The QRS complex corresponds to the ventricles contracting
- The T wave is repolarization

Resting EKG
For a resting EKG, position the patient lying down, face up.
- If the patient has difficulty breathing (dyspnea), prop the patient's head up with pillows
- For a stress test, 12—15 leads are attached to the patient, who runs on a treadmill
- For a Holter monitor, 3—5 leads are used, and the results of the EKG are recorded on a telemetry device worn around the patient's neck for 24—48 hours

EKG interpretation
A normal sinus rhythm (NSR) on an EKG denotes that the electrical impulses start in the sinoatrial node (SA) first, and cause the right and left atria to contract simultaneously to effectively pump blood into the ventricles. The contraction of the atria is followed by contraction of the ventricles, which move blood throughout the body. The conduction system coordinates the contractions. If the SA node does not initiate the electrical impulse, the atrioventricular node (AV) can do so.

The AV node is not as capable of increasing the heart rate as is the SA node, because the AV resting rate is lower than that of the SA node. The patient requires a mechanical pacemaker to fix the slow heart rate. All of the cells of the heart are capable of generating the electrical impulses necessary to trigger a heartbeat; this property is known as automaticity. Signal conduction problems, termed block, can occur at any site along the conduction pathway, causing an arrhythmia, which is an alteration in the normal rhythm.

Aneroid sphygmomanometer

Blood pressure is measured as systolic and diastolic pressure by means of a stethoscope and an aneroid sphygmomanometer (portable blood pressure cuff). For example, if the reading is 120/80 mm/Hg, 120 is the systole, and 80 is the diastole. The first Korotkoff sound the CMA hears is the systole; the last Korotkoff sound is the diastole.

- Position the blood pressure cuff so that it surrounds 75% of the patient's upper arm
- The width of the cuff bladder should exceed the diameter of the patient's arm by 20% or more
- This is about 40% of the circumference of the arm
- Fit the cuff so that the bottom edge sits about one inch above the elbow joint
- Place the stethoscope's diaphragm over the patient's radial artery, and insert the earpieces into your ears
- Inflate the cuff quickly, in 7 seconds or less
- Deflate the blood pressure cuff slowly, at a rate of 2—3 mm/Hg per second
- Remove the cuff and stethoscope
- Record the measurement in your patient's chart immediately

Blood pressure

Increased blood pressure contributes to stroke and heart disease. Low blood pressure is associated with shock, trauma, bleeding, or severe infection.

Upper normal adult blood pressure: 120/80 mm/Hg (millimeters of mercury)
Prehypertension: Systole between 120 and 139 and diastole between 80 and 90
Borderline hypertension (high blood pressure): 140/90 mm/Hg
Hypertension Stage 1: Systole between 140 and 159 and diastole between 90 and 99
Hypertension Stage 2: Systole 160 or more and diastole of 100 or more
Hypotension (low blood pressure): 90/50 mm/Hg or less

False BP results can occur from:
- Incorrect cuff size — If your patient is obese, use a thigh cuff on the upper arm. If your patient is a child, use a pediatric cuff
- Deflating the cuff more rapidly than 2—3 mm/Hg per second
- Venous congestion makes it difficult to hear the blood pressure sounds. Elevating the patient's arm after positioning the cuff but before inflating it can decrease venous congestion
- Loud environmental noises
- Operator error

Body temperature

A live patient's body temperature is measured to determine if he/she is storing and releasing heat properly, to detect abnormally high or low body temperatures, and to assess the effectiveness of some types of medications. The coroner measures temperature to determine time of death. Human temperature ranges are:

- Ideal 98.6°F (37°C)
- Normal Range 97.8°F (36.5°C) — 99°F (37.2°C)
- Hypothermia (too cold) <95°F (<35°C)
- Pyrexia (fever) >98.6°F oral or >99.8°F rectal
- Hyperpyrexia (lethal fever) 107.6°F (>42°C)

Temperature is lowest around 4:00 a.m. and highest around 6:00 p.m.

- Temperature spikes occur after meals
- Ovulation in women creates a temperature rise of 0.5°F—1°F when measured before arising from bed in the morning (basal body temperature)
- Individual temperature differences in healthy people are due to the rate of metabolism
- Patients with hypothyroidism tend to be cold
- Body temperature differs at different sites
- Normal oral temperature is 98.6 °F, while normal rectal temperature is 99.6 °F (37.6°C)
- The mouth is open to the air, so its temperature is lower
- Do not take the patient's oral temperature for 30 minutes after eating or drinking, as it will be raised with hot food, and decreased with cold drinks

Nebulizer therapy

A Nebulizer is a therapeutic device that allows the patient to inhale medication in mist form.

- The purpose of nebulizer treatments is to alleviate difficulty breathing (dyspnea) associated with lung diseases such as asthma, emphysema, lung cancer, and Chronic Obstructive Pulmonary Disease (COPD)
- Examples of nebulizer medication are Pulmicort Repsules (budesonide) and Atrovent (ipratropium)
- You must check the regulations in the state in which you practice, as some states do not permit CMAs to administer medication
- Assist the Registered Nurse in nebulizer administration by preparing the patient for treatment
- Position the patient, clean and assemble the nebulizer apparatus, and encouraging the patient in deep breathing and coughing exercises prior to and after treatment
- Recognize side-effects of nebulizer therapy, like slow clinical response that can require a switch to IV

Quest. 48 place face mask over the patients mouth and nose to make sure the majority of medication is inhaled. Patient should take deep breaths.

Pulse oximetry

Pulse oximetry non-invasively measures a patient's oxyhemoglobin level during stress tests or emergency medicine, which is much easier for the patient than having painful arterial blood gases (SaO2) drawn at intervals.

- Use a pulse oximeter to monitor your at-risk patient's oxygen saturation level (SpO2) continuously
- Attach the oximeter sensor to one of the patient's first three fingers (index, middle or ring)
- If the patient's hands are damaged, use a toe or earlobe
- Consider using the forehead, nose, or other parts of the foot only as a last resort
- It should always read between 95% and 100%
- An alarm sounds if the SpO2 falls under 90% -- tell the doctor the patient is hypoxic
- Many oximeters also give the patient's heart rate at the same time
- A pulse oximeter is not accurate if the patient is very anemic, has poor circulation, is edematous, moves a lot, or wears artificial nails or very dark nail polish
- Adjust the room temperature, lighting, and move electronic equipment to get a good reading

Patient preparation & assisting the physician

Trendelenburg

Also known as shock position, where the patient is supine (face up) with the feet elevated and the head down.
- If your patient faints when you draw his/her blood, then place him/her in a left side-lying

Trendelenburg position to increase blood flow to the brain and reverse syncope)
- Place a patient with an air embolism from an IV in the Trendelenburg position to decrease the chance that the embolism will push further into the pulmonary circulation

Sims

Sims is a left side-lying position that often benefits the patient suffering with abdominal distension or ascites from liver disease.

Orthopneic

Orthopneic is also known as the semi-Fowler position; the patient is seated upright and leaning forward to allow easy respiration. Avoid placing a patient with breathing difficulty (dyspnea) in the supine position (reclining on the back). The orthopneic position is good for EKG patients with labored breathing to minimize artifacts on the tracing.

Patient education techniques

Age	Learning Issue	Teaching Solution
Infant	Non-verbal	Teach the parents or guardian
Preschooler	Short attention span	Instruct with visuals (e.g., dolls) and role play Tell parents to oversee treatment
5 to 8 yrs.	Longer attention span and eager for knowledge	Use short videos, visuals, and pictures
9 to 12 yrs.	Good attention span, great curiosity, and some independence. Rapid growth issues, such as mixed dentition. Desire for group acceptance.	Teach pairs or small groups, if confidentiality can be preserved Use age-appropriate language to indicate respect
13 to 15 yrs.	Peer pressure; personal appearance; poor coordination; bad eating habits	Give individualized instructions, motivation and encouragement
16 to 19 yrs.	Question authority; have busy schedules	Act as a friend and mentor. Explain disease process and anatomy.
20 to 60 yrs.	Individualized problems	Tailor instruction to the individual circumstances, e.g., pregnancy, depression, drug abuse
60+ yrs.	Age-related problems (e.g., eyesight, memory, mobility, multiple prescriptions); fixed income; isolation; dependence on caregiver	Educate caregivers and patient. Emphasize avoiding triggers. Dispense free samples (promotions from suppliers). Register patient with wandering registry, if necessary.

Patient's own equipment

Discourage patients from bringing their own equipment into your facility. Examples of patient-owned equipment are CPAP machines, pain pumps, wheelchairs, heaters, fans, hairdryers, televisions, and coffee pots. Even though the equipment is for personal use, it still represents a risk to your facility because it may:

- Not meet high safety standards (e.g., NFPA, JCAHO)
- Contain infectious agents or vermin
- Be used in an unsafe manner (e.g., the patient may have bypassed safety alarms)

When your patient brings his/her own equipment into the facility for regular, extended use, then you must contact Engineering for an incoming inspection.

- An engineer evaluates the device for fire safety, alarm functionality and audibility, and cleanliness
- The engineer will need a copy of the operating manual and will affix a numbered sticker on the equipment for tracking and service
- Your Risk Manager will probably disallow life-support devices, such as ventilators, due to liability issues
- The patient must be alert and capable of operating personal equipment in a safe manner

Patients own medications

Your patient may bring his/her own medications into your facility for self-administration, for example, an Epi-pen, asthma puffer, insulin, pain pump, or nitroglycerin.

- This means your patient gets instant treatment, but it also represents a liability to the facility
- The drugs could be improperly stored, shared, stolen, or mistakenly administered to another patient
- The syringes used to administer the medication may be disposed of incorrectly in the regular garbage, instead of a sharps safe, and present a hazard to cleaning staff

The CMA may assist the patient with self-administration to the extent of:

- Checking the label and dosage to ensure it is taken as directed
- Opening the case and placing the medication in the patient's hand
- Ensuring safe disposal of sharps (e.g., broken ampoules, needles)
- However, you may not actually inject or otherwise administer the medication without the doctor's express instructions
- Your liability is greatest for medications marked "as needed" (prn)
- Most states require caregivers to take a 4-hour training course with a pharmacist or registered nurse before allowing medication assistance

Patient history interview

A patient history is a written record gathered from a patient interview,

listing past and present health, family information, and personal information pertinent to health, such as occupation. A History and Physical Examination Report (H&P) is a single report with two segments. It is usually dictated and transcribed, but can be a form. The Joint Commission requires an H&P within 24 hours of admission for acute care patients and within 30 days prior to admission for chronic care patients. This must then be updated within 24 hours after the patient is admitted.

A Medical History and Review of System form the basis for the provisional diagnosis and treatment plan. The doctor collects information from the patient, guardian, or a reliable source (e.g., ambulance attendant or personal support worker). The headings are:

- Chief Complaint
- Symptoms
- History of Present Illness
- Medical History
- Family History
- Social History
- Health Maintenance
- Review of Systems

The Joint Commission requires minors to have a developmental age evaluation and educational needs assessment, also.

Collecting and processing specimens

Venipuncture equipment

Routine adult venipuncture equipment:
- Completed requisition with a physician's signature and billing information
- Soap, water, and towels for hand washing
- Sufficient evacuated blood tubes with the right color stopper
- One 21g or 22g cannula X 1.5" length
- Plastic Vacutainer holder with a luer-lock hub
- Isopropyl alcohol or povidone-iodine swab
- Clean, dry cotton balls
- Band-aid or Micropore tape, if the patient is allergic to adhesive
- Tourniquet (rubber Penrose catheter or blood pressure cuff)
- Kidney basin or tray to hold the specimen during collection
- Latex or vinyl gloves
- Pen with indelible ink
- Plastic biohazard bag with outer pouch for the requisition
- Well-buttoned lab coat to protect your clothing
- Reclining chair or bed to support the patient
- Certain tests require chemical additives, ice, or a hot water bath
- Sharps disposal container
- Garbage can

The patient identification and consent procedures that is legally required before attempting venipuncture:
- If the patient requires an interpreter, get one
- Identify yourself to the patient
- Tell the patient which doctor requested the blood sample
- Explain in general terms what you are going to do
- Check the patient's armband or health card to confirm identity
- Verify the correct spelling of the patient's name and date of birth
- If there is any discrepancy between the patient's written identification and your requisition, STOP. Get a doctor or nurse who knows the patient to confirm the identity, and note this on the requisition
- A conscious, adult patient has the right to refuse treatment. If you proceed with collection after the patient has refused it, you can be charged with battery. Mark "*PATIENT REFUSED*" with your initials, the date and time on the requisition, return it to the patient's chart, and inform the charge nurse at once. If the patient is unconscious, the law considers you have been given implied consent

The preparation steps for venipuncture:
- Check the expiration dates on all tubes, cannulae and swabs. Get fresh products if any have expired
- Wash, dry, and glove your hands

- 75 -

- Place the equipment in the kidney basin on an easily accessible table, not on the bed where they can break if the patient rolls over
- Select the patient's arm that has no intravenous fluid drip or injury
- Tie the tourniquet around the patient's bicep, or inflate a blood pressure cuff to 20 mm/Hg
- Ask the patient to clench a fist. Palpate the veins in the ante cubital fossa
- If the arm turns blue, or if the patient complains the tourniquet is too tight, loosen it immediately. Wait until the arm returns to a normal color before reapplying. Prolonged or repeated use of the tourniquet or blood pressure cuff can result in artificially high calcium levels in the specimen

Draw blood via venipuncture

Position the patient's arm on a pillow so blood flows downwards. Tell the patient to remain still.
- Retract the skin from the site, so it does not clog the bevel
- Uncap the 21 or 22 gauge cannula
- Rest the first tube inside the holder
- Do not push it onto the hub. Insert the cannula, bevel up, into the vein at a 30° angle
- Grasp the holder with one hand
- Push the tube onto the hub with the other

- Blood flows automatically into the evacuated tube when the stopper is pierced, and stops when its vacuum is depleted
- Detach the filled tube from the end of the cannula. Invert the tube several times to mix the anticoagulant and blood
- Place the filled tube in the kidney basin
- Release the tourniquet to relax the pressure, so blood does not spurt when you remove the cannula from the patient's arm. Rest cotton over the puncture site
- Remove the cannula while still on the end of its holder, without unscrewing it
- Apply steady pressure to the wound for 4 to 6 minutes to stop bleeding – longer if the patient is taking anticoagulant drugs like aspirin or Coumadin
- Ask the alert patient to continue applying pressure after the first minute, so you can dispose of the used equipment
- Elevate the puncture slightly to help slow bleeding, but do not bend the arm
- Apply a band-aid

Routine urinalysis according to the tests on an N-Multistix.

Below are the common urine dipstick tests in routine urinalysis. Normal values are bracketed:
- *Blood (negative)*: Intact or hemolyzed red blood cells indicate bleeding due to infection, menstruation,

paroxysmal hemoglobinuria, or trauma

- *Glucose (negative):* Uncontrolled diabetes and women with gestational diabetes spill sugar into their urine when their renal threshold is exceeded
- *Ketones (negative):* Uncontrolled diabetes, extreme dieters, and starving people produce ketones in urine when their bodies burn fat instead of sugar
- *Leukocytes (negative):* White blood cells indicate bleeding due to infection
- *pH (5 to 9):* Acidic urine helps the bladder resist infection. Alkaline urine encourages bacterial growth
- *Protein (up to 8 mg/dl):* Albumin is shed from the kidneys if the nephrons are damaged. Trace protein can be from genitals or feces
- *Nitrites (negative):* Some bacteria, like E-coli, produce nitrites after eating nitrates, so this is an indicator of infection

If kidney stones, infection, or damage are suspected, then a microscopic urinalysis is performed with the routine urinalysis (R&M) for casts, crystals, and cells. Routine urinalysis according to the tests on an N-Multistix.

Blood collection by capillary puncture

Capillary puncture is suitable when a very small quantity of blood is required and the patient has difficult veins. Examples of when capillary puncture is appropriate include:

- Newborn PKU
- Diabetic glucose via glucometer
- Anemic hemoglobin via hemoglobinometer
- Bleeding time before surgery

Capillary puncture is inappropriate for blood cultures or large quantities because the site clots quickly.

- Perform newborn capillary puncture with a short point lancet on the lateral or medial plantar heel surface to avoid nicking the calcaneous (heel bone) and causing osteomyelitis
- The infant may require a foot amputation if the site becomes gangrenous
- Older infants can have the plantar surface of their big toes pricked with a short point lancet
- Children and adults have the distal phalanx palmar surface pricked with a long point lancet

Collecting blood by capillary puncture correctly:

- Wash the puncture site with warm water to dilate capillaries.
- If the site remains cold, apply a chemical warming pack, such as Hot Shots used by skiers in their gloves
- Wrap the pack in a cloth so it does not directly contact the infant's thin skin
- Swab the site with alcohol
- Puncture the skin quickly with a lancet

- Draw blood into the Microtainer tube by capillary action and GENTLE squeezing in this order:

Color	Additive	Order of Draw	# of Inversions
Dark Green	Lithium Heparin	Second	Mix 10 times
Gold and Amber	SST	Fourth	Do not mix
Lavender	EDTA	First	Mix 20 times
Mint Green	PST	Third	Mix 10 times
Red	None	Last	Do not mix

The order of draw is different than that used for venipuncture because capillary blood is more likely to clot or hemolyze during collection.

- Wiping the puncture with alcohol to encourage bleeding when the wound has already clotted will dilute the specimen
- Vigorous squeezing can cause interstitial fluid to leak into the specimen and dilute it, or hemolysis of red blood cells, giving a false result

O&P and pinworm stool collection

Stool for ova and parasites (O&P) means the lab looks for worms (helminthes) and protozoa that can cause anemia in feces samples, such as tapeworm and round worms. Give the patient a clean jar containing an ounce of formalin. Tell the patient to use a popsicle stick to mix a teaspoon of stool with the preservative and return it, tightly capped and labeled, to the lab.

Pinworms are white, thread-like parasites usually contracted by children from sand boxes in which infected cats and dogs have defecated. The child often scratches his/her itchy bottom and grinds the teeth while sleeping. Give the parent a stool container containing a pinworm paddle, or tell the parent to use a jar with clear tape.

- When the child sleeps, use a flashlight to visualize the anus
- Female tapeworms leave the bowel to lay eggs around the anus at night
- Gently touch the paddle or tape to the anus and place it in the jar
- Cap tightly. Wash hands well. Return the labeled jar to the lab

Occult blood and guaiac stool collection

Patients who use Aspirin regularly or have ulcers may lose microscopic amounts of blood in their feces. The lab examines stool smears on a mail-in card for occult blood. Give your patient an occult blood kit.

- Tell him or her to follow the enclosed diet for three days before collection, as foods that cause bleeding must be avoided (e.g., cantaloupe, turnip, broccoli and horseradish).
- Tell the patient to place plastic wrap under the toilet seat and defecate
- Use the enclosed popsicle sticks to smear thin samples of stool from three consecutive bowel movements on the three windows in the card

- The patient mails the card back to the lab in the envelope provided

Guaiac also detects occult blood, but is collected by the doctor in the office during a rectal examination with a gloved finger.
- The doctor wipes the soiled glove across a window that contains guaiac resin on a card and adds two drops of peroxide
- If the sample oxidizes (turns blue) in 2 seconds or less, the patient is losing blood

These two tests are not reliable for bowel cancer.

Plate a specimen for C&S

Sensitivity testing is also called culture and susceptibility testing (C&S).
- Wash your hands
- Don gloves and a lab coat
- Sterilize a loop
- Streak body fluid (stool, urine, blood, sputum, or wound drainage) across an agar plate with the loop
- Rotate the loop and streak again so the bacteria are evenly distributed across the agar
- You may also place tissue on media. Incubate at body temperature (37°C) for 24 to 48 hours

If growth occurs, the lab distinguishes normal flora from pathogens by chemical and enzyme tests. A lab tech inoculates pathogens with antimicrobials to see if they can be killed (susceptible), or cannot be killed (resistant). If the antimicrobial that works best requires high doses (intermediate), it is likely to be toxic to the patient. The doctor initially prescribes the antimicrobial to which the pathogen is susceptible, except if the patient is allergic to it. The doctor consults with a pharmacist and microbiologist to choose the least toxic alternative, but the intermediate dose may need to be given over a long time and the patient may suffer side-effects. If the pathogen is resistant to many antimicrobials, then expensive intravenous combination therapy may be the only effective treatment.

Sputum culture collection

Sputum is phlegm (mucous) and other matter expelled from the lungs and trachea. It should contain as little saliva from the mouth as possible. Sputum can be cultured (C&S) to identify an infection, such as pneumonia. Sputum can be examined microscopically to identify cancer or a disease-causing agent, such as asbestos fibers. If the doctor orders sputum for AFB (acid fast bacilli stain), then the lab searches for bacteria that cause tuberculosis.
- Drink fluids the night before specimen collection, to encourage secretions
- Collect the specimen upon arising, because sputum collects in the air passageways during sleep
- Tap on the chest
- Cough deeply
- If you cannot produce any sputum, try inhaling steaming salt water

- If any sputum arises, spit it into a sterile cup
- Cap it tightly and label it
- Bring the sputum to the lab immediately for testing
- If you cannot transport it immediately, refrigerate it up to 3 days
- Sometimes the doctor orders specimen collection on 3 consecutive days
- The patient should be instructed to drink fluids the night before specimen collection to encourage secretions
- The specimen should be collected upon arising because sputum collects in the air passageway during sleep
- The chest should be tapped and the patient should be instructed to cough deeply
- If sputum is not produced, the patient should be instructed to try inhaling steaming salt water
- If any sputum arises, the patient should be instructed to spit it into a sterile cup
- The cup should be capped tightly and labeled

Centers for Disease Control guidelines
When the CMA encounters a doctor's order to collect, ship, or store an unfamiliar specimen or vaccine, then he/she should visit the Web site for the Centers for Disease Control at http://emergency.cdc.gov/labissues/#shipping. Scroll through the alphabetical lists of infectious agents and chemical terrorism agents. The CDC's charts briefly explain how to safely collect, store, plate, stain and

transport dangerous biological materials. Often, the CDC also estimates the patient's chance of recovery.

Your employer may decide to use dangerous biological agents and toxins for research. If these materials are a serious threat to human, animal or plant life, then you must register them with the National Select Agent Registry. Obtain the necessary registration forms and advice at http://www.selectagents.gov/index.html

QA manager

Your facility must comply with The Joint Commission's Standards Improvement Initiative to obtain accreditation. If your facility treats Medicare patients, then it must also comply with:
- The federal Healthcare Quality Improvement Program (HCQIP)
- Quality Improvement Organization (QIO) projects
- Quality Improvement System for Managed Care (QISMC)
- Your facility may want the prestige associated with the International Standards Organization (ISO) standard for quality management (9001:2000)
- The Quality Assurance (QA) Manager ensures your facility follows best practices required by these standards
- The QA Manager uses tracer methodology to ensure the quality of patient care is excellent

- 80 -

- Help the QA Manager with data collection when asked

Safety officer

The Safety Officer arranges for your safety training at your employer's expense and informs you of pertinent changes OSHA makes. The Safety Officer checks waste disposal of radioactive, infectious and chemically contaminated items. The Safety Officer devises a computerized error reporting system, focused on process rather than individuals and punitive actions, and reviews errors to find trends and patterns. The Safety Officer establishes rapid response teams and investigates adverse incidents.

Hemodialysis patient manual hemoglobin test

Test the hemoglobinometer with known controls first.
- Polish a clean hemocytometer slide with lens paper
- Fill a blue-ringed, unheparinized capillary tube with blood
- Place one drop of blood on the hemocytometer slide
- Roll the heparinized, wooden hemolysis stick over the blood drop until the blood is hemolyzed and transparent (about 30 seconds)
- Place the cover slip over the slide
- Slide them together into the hemoglobinometer
- Look through the viewer
- Adjust the light until the two fields you see are exactly the same color (Most

hemoglobinometers use green and black).
- Read the scale (usually on the side of the meter) and record the hemoglobin level. (Normal values are 12—16 g/dl for women, and 14—16 g/dl for men)
- Disassemble the slide and cover slip
- Sanitize, disinfect, polish, and case them
- Wipe the test area and outside of the hemoglobinometer with disinfectant
- Hemoglobinometer readings with capillary blood show about 10% false-positives for anemia, as compared to venous Coulter Counter readings
- Hemoglobinometers are for point-of-care testing for "ballpark" estimates

Hematocrit test

A hematocrit (Hct) test separates the blood cells from the plasma in a centrifuge as part of a complete blood count (CBC). Hct indirectly measures red blood cell (RBC) mass, so if the RBCs are of normal size, then the Hct should confirm the RBC count. Patients with macrocytic, microcytic, or iron deficiency anemia with small RBCs will not have parallel Hct and RBC counts. Report results as Packed Cell Volume (PCV), meaning the percentage by volume of packed red blood cells in whole blood. Normal values for venous blood are:
- Males 42% to 52%
- Females 36% to 48%

- Microhematocrit readings from capillary tubes are a little higher
- Babies have higher hematocrits than adults because they have more macrocytic RBC's
- An abnormal hematocrit suggests follow-up tests must be done for a firm diagnosis.

Low hematocrit readings (less than 30%) may indicate many diseases:
- Adrenal insufficiency, anemia, burns, Hodgkin's disease, leukemia, or poisoning
- High hematocrit can be from erythrocytosis, polycythemia vera or shock

ESR

An erythrocyte sedimentation rate (ESR or sed rate) measures how far blood cells with anticoagulant (EDTA or sodium citrate) will fall in a clump (aggregate) in a Westergren or Wintrobe tube in one hour, due to changes in plasma proteins (Rouleaux formation). Normal RBC's do not form Rouleaux, and they settle slowly. Normal values are:
- Males 0—15 millimeters per hour
- Females 0—20 mm/h
- Children 0—10 mm/h
- RBC settling for patients over 50 years old may normally measure 5—10 mm/h more

If RBC's settle quickly, the Rouleaux indicates some type of inflammation, necrosis, or parasites are present and further tests are required, but a sed rate does not definitively diagnose a disease. A high ESR can indicate many

diseases: Anemia, arthritis, cancer, heart attack, lupus, pelvic inflammatory disease, kidney disease, pneumonia, poisoning with heavy metals, syphilis, thyroid disease, toxemia, tuberculosis. A low sed rate can be from heavy blood loss.

Normal values for RBC, WBC, and platelets

The CMA performs a quality control test on the Coulter Counter every 8 hours by manually comparing RBC, WBC and platelet counts on a smear against the machine's reading for the same patient. The patient's blood may be normal, but the machine could report an incorrect result if the quality of the stain used was poor (too acid or alkali), the specimen was diluted incorrectly, or the machine's calculation was inaccurate.

Test	Normal Values
RBC count	Babies 4.8 to 7.2 million cells per microliter of blood (cells/mcL) Adult males 4.7 to 6.1 million cells/mcL Adult females 4 to 5 million cells/mcL , but lower in pregnancy
WBC count	4,500 to 10,000 WBC's per microliter in total (cells/mcL) Differential is: 1% basophils; 1 to 3% eosinophils; neutrophils 50% to 70%; lymphocytes 15 to 40%; and monocytes 2 to 8%.
Platelets	Babies 200,000 to 475,000 per microliter of blood (x 106/Liter) Adults 150,000 to 450,000 (x 106/Liter)

Patients taking coumadin

The three tests used to monitor patients who take the blood thinner (anticoagulant) coumadin are INR, PT, and PTT. Note that PT and PTT are being phased out in favor of INR.

- INR (international normalized ratio) checks clotting Factor VII to I. It standardizes different tissue factors (thromboplastin) used worldwide for testing. Normal INR is 0.9—1.2. If a patient has an INR under 2.0, there is little bleeding. If a patient has an INR of 3.0—4.5, there is heavy bleeding (hemorrhage). Most patients on anticoagulant therapy (coumadin, heparin, and warfarin) are kept with an INR of 2.0 to 3.0, depending on their condition. If the patient is very likely to develop blood clots, the doctor may push the INR to 3.5. Therapeutic INR is checked every 4—6 weeks. Prolonged INR may be due to bile deficiency, cirrhosis of the liver, lack of Vitamin K, or small intestine disease
- Normal PT (prothrombin time) is 10—12 seconds. Therapeutic value is 13—18 seconds. PT checks Factor VII to I
- Normal PTT (partial thromboplastin time) is 25—38 seconds. Therapeutic value is 38—76 seconds. PTT checks Factor XII to I

Biochemistry tests

The purpose of the following Biochemistry tests:

- All four tests monitor blood sugar for suspected or confirmed diabetes
- *Fasting blood sugar*: Tell the patient to fast 8 hours before collection. Do not drink excessive water, as it dilutes the sugar. Normal fasting value is less than 110mg/dl. Use a grey stoppered tube because the oxalate preservative stops the blood cells from eating sugar
- *2 hr. p.c.*: Two hours post cibum (after eating). After the fasting blood collection, the patient takes a normal meal and returns for a second collection exactly 2 hours after it was finished. Blood sugar should peak two hours after eating (postprandial), and then drop precipitously
- *Hb A1c:* A test for glucose bound to hemoglobin in red blood cells over their 120-day lifespan. It is a snapshot of blood glucose control for the past three months and can help to evaluate the effectiveness of strategies being used to control diabetes such as medication or diet
- *GTT*: A 3 or 5 hour glucose tolerance test diagnoses hyperglycemia (high blood sugar) that is a precursor to diabetes. Collect blood and urine fasting, 30 minute after a glucose drink was finished, and at 1 hour, 2 hours, and 3 hours. Occasionally it is ordered at 4 and 5 hours

Kidney function tests

Kidney (renal) function tests and their normal values:

- *BUN:* Blood Urea Nitrogen (BUN) is a nitrogenous waste by-product of amino acid metabolism. Urea is the end product. BUN is normally excreted by the kidneys at 7—18 mg/dL. Patients with end-stage renal disease (ESRD) have BUN levels between 60—100 mg/dL, and are monitored monthly
- *Creatinine:* Creatinine is the end-product of muscle metabolism and is normally removed by the kidneys at 0.7 to 1.5 mg/dl. High creatinine (over 1.5 mg/dl) and BUN (over 20 mg/dl) means the patient has a kidney disease (e.g., glomerulonephritis, pyelonephritis, stones, tubular necrosis, or tumors)
- *Protein:* A normal serum protein test includes Total Protein 6 to 8 g/dl, Albumin 3.2 to 4.5 g/dl, and Globulin 2.3 to 3.4 g/dl. Albumin deficiency causes swelling (edema) and can be from protein malnutrition, kidney or liver, and disease. Low globulin indicates severe burns, malnutrition, kidney or liver disease
- *Urea:* Carbamide, a nitrogenous waste product of protein metabolism made by the liver from ammonia and aspartic acid (an amino acid). Healthy kidneys eliminate 50 g of urea daily. Purified urea is used as a diuretic, pressure reducer, and antiseptic

Liver function tests

The liver function tests and their normal values:

- ALP (Alkaline Phosphatase) normally ranges from 30 to 85 IU/L (International Units/liter)adults and up to 300 in children with growing bones. Doctors use ALP to differentiate between bone and liver diseases. ALP increases in bone fractures and Paget's disease, liver cancer, hyperparathyroidism, hyperphosphatasia, infarcted bowel, and rheumatoid arthritis. ALP decreases in pernicious anemia, celiac disease, hypothyroidism, low serum phosphorous (hypophosphatemia), and malnutrition
- ALT (Serum Alanine Aminotransferase) normally ranges from 5 to 35 IU/L. ALT increases in liver disease. AST: ALT ratio should be 1:1. If it is greater than 1:1, it can mean cirrhosis, congestion, or tumors of the liver. If the ratio is less than 1:1, suspect hepatitis or mononucleosis
- AST (Serum Aspartate Aminotransferase) normally ranges from 5 to 40 IU/L. AST increases in conditions that affect the heart such as congestive heart failure, liver such as chronic alcohol or drug abuse or cirrhosis, muscles

such as muscular dystrophy, or pancreatitis
- Bilirubin normally ranges from 1.7 to 5.1 ғmol/L. It is a reddish-yellow bile pigment created when the liver breaks down old red blood cells, and is stored in the gall bladder. Excess bilirubin causes jaundice. The CMA can artificially lower bilirubin by leaving a specimen tube exposed to light at room temperature for one hour, shaking the specimen, or allowing air bubbles in it.

Lipid profile

A lipid profile tests for hyperlipidemia, elevated fats and oils in the blood, which clog blood vessels and result in heart attack, stroke, and ischemia. Routinely screen men over 35, women over 45, and younger patients with risk factors or a significant family history of cardiovascular disease.

Lipid	Normal Value
LDL cholesterol (bad cholesterol)	Above 160 mg/dL High 130-159 mg/dl borderline high 100-129 mg/dl near optimal <100 mg/dl is optimal
HDL cholesterol (good cholesterol)	>40 mg/dl male > 50 mg/dl female
Total cholesterol	< 200 mg/dl is desirable 200-239 mg/dL is borderline high risk 240 mg/dL and above is high risk
LDL/HDL ratio	<4
Triglycerides	< 150 mg/dL normal 150-199 mg/dL borderline high Above 200 mg/dL is considered high

Tell your patient to fast 12 to 14 hours before testing. Random lipids are inaccurate because fatty meals spike them. Treatment is diet modification, exercise, weight loss, niacin supplements, statins for cholesterol (Lipitor, Mevacor), and fibrates for triglyceride (Lopid, Tricor).

Mononucleosis test

Epstein-Barr virus (EBV) causes mononucleosis. The Monospot heterophile antibodies test confirms the patient is in the early stage of mononucleosis (2—9 weeks).
- To perform a Monospot, drop capillary or venous blood on a glass slide
- Mix with guinea pig kidney antigen to absorb Forssmann antibodies
- Mix with beef red blood stroma to absorb non-Forssman antibodies
- Mix with horse blood
- Guinea pig agglutination means the patient has early mononucleosis
- Beef should not agglutinate
- Monospot can be false-negative on children under 10, or before two weeks of infection
- False-positives are caused by adenovirus, Burkitt's and Hodgkin's lymphomas, cytomegalovirus, hepatitis, HIV, leukemia, lupus, pregnancy, rheumatoid arthritis, rubella, and toxoplasmosis
- Monospot may not detect infection older than six months

If your patient has late stage mono, the doctor orders EBV antibody titer, CBC, and throat swab.
- To perform a titer, serially dilute blood serum or other body fluids with saline
- Negative is less than 1:40 EBV and no IgM antibodies are present
- Positive is greater than 1:40 and antibodies are present. IgM indicates the active phase of mono. IgG antibodies mean the patient is recovering from mononucleosis

Strep test

Often, acute pharyngitis results from Group A Streptococci. Strep throat especially affects children 5 to 15 years old in the winter and spring. Strep throat can develop into rheumatic fever when it travels through the bloodstream to destroy the heart, joints, and kidneys. Super Strep is resistant to antibiotics.

To perform a Quidel QuickVue rapid strep test:
- Swab the patient's tonsils and pharynx for no more than 5 seconds with the swab in the kit
- Use a tongue depressor to avoid swabbing the cheeks and tongue
- The patient will gag briefly
- Place the swab in the test cassette chamber
- Crush the extraction reagent delivery device
- Mix the extraction solutions until they turn green

- Add the solution to the top rim of the swab chamber
- Stand the swab upright in the chamber so capillary action draws the solution up to the rabbit reagent pad
- Read the window at 5 minutes
- A red stripe on the reagent strip indicates strep infection
- The control is the blue line next to the letter C, and it should always appear
- The absence of a red line indicates no strep infection
- A positive result means the patient requires antibiotic treatment to avoid rheumatic fever

C-reactive protein

C-reactive protein (CRP) is a globulin required to resist bacterial infections and inflammation. CRP binds to dying cells to activate the complement system, triggering it to fight infection and disease. Young people normally have a CRP less than 10 mg/L. Pregnant women, the elderly, and patients with mild viral infections or inflammation have a slightly elevated CRP of 10 to 40 mg/L. However, CRP rises in 6 hours after a severe infection or inflammation occurs, up to 200 mg/L. People with massive burns or overwhelming bacterial infections have CRP levels over 200 mg/L. CRP peaks in 48 hours. CRP is elevated in patients with rheumatic fever, heart disease, colon cancer, pneumonia, tuberculosis, lupus, diabetes, vasculitis, rheumatoid arthritis, septic arthritis, and osteomyelitis. Athletes who train too much decrease their CRP and become more susceptible to infections, as a result. Draw 10 ml of blood in a red stoppered tube. The Immunohistochemistry lab performs an ELISA latex agglutination test to find C-reactive protein. A positive result indicates only inflammation somewhere in the body.

Pregnancy testing

Beta Human Chorionic Gonadotropin (beta- HCG) is the substance the lab tests urine or blood for to confirm female pregnancy or gestational tumors, or testicular tumors in males. It is performed preoperatively as a precaution for women of childbearing age.

Qualitative hCG just confirms the pregnancy, as it is detectable one week after conception.
- Tell your patient to collect the first morning urine sample, if possible, because it is most concentrated
- Avoid taking diuretics or the antihistamine promethazine, because it could create a false-negative result
- Tell the doctor if you took drugs to control epilepsy or Parkinson's disease, or tranquilizers or hypnotics to induce sleep because they can cause false-positive results
- At least 50 ml is required in a clean jar
- The specimen must not be contaminated with stool, menstrual blood, semen, or prostate extractions

Quantitative hCG helps diagnose ectopic or failing pregnancy, ovarian or testicular tumors, or monitors a woman after a miscarriage.
- Draw a red stoppered tube of blood for the lab
- High levels of Beta hCG in blood indicate tumor progression
- Low levels indicate effective cancer treatment

Gram-negative bacteria

Thin-walled bacteria that turns RED when Gram stained from absorbing crystal violet, pink safrinin, and fuchsin. Lipopolysaccharide in their walls repels blue stain. Lipid-A is the endotoxin found outside the cell wall. Parts include: Flagellum (motility); pilus (adherence, conjugation); capsule (protection); peptidoglycan wall (support, shape); cytoplasmic membrane; and periplasmic space (holds enzymes and proteins). Examples: Escherichia coli; Klebsiella pneumoniae; Pseudomonas aeruginosa; Haemophilus influenzae; Enterobacter aerogenes.

Gram-positive bacteria

Thick-walled bacteria that turns VIOLET-BLUE when Gram stained. Walls contain teichoic acid and a membrane that increase virulence. Examples: Group B Streptococcus; Staphylococcus aureus and epidermidis; Listeria monocytogenes. Most bone infections (osteomyelitis) are caused by Gram-positive bacteria.

Virus

Virus is a tiny infectious agent only 20 to 300 nm across that needs a living host to reproduce. A virus has a protein coat, an RNA or DNA nucleus, and sometimes an envelope. More fragile than bacteria and lose infectivity quickly when removed from their host. Examples: HIV, rubella, and influenza.

Bacteria

Bacteria is a primitive, single-celled microorganism with no membraned nucleus (prokaryotic), measuring 0.1 ᶠ m to 10 ᶠm. Bacteria have a cytoplasm center, covered by a cell wall made of protein and complex carbohydrates. Bacteria can be free-living, parasites (living on a live host), or saprophytic (living on decaying matter). They reproduce quickly and waste products cause disease. Bacteria are transported by animals, plants, wind, and water. Examples: Tuberculosis, salmonella, and campylobacter.

Fungus

Fungus is a plant-like, single-celled microorganisms with a rigid cell wall, measuring 8 ᶠm to 10 mm. Fungi have no green chlorophyll, and include lichen, mildews, molds, mushrooms, rusts, smuts, and yeasts. Fungi decompose organic matter by absorbing nutrients through hyphae and mycelium. Examples: Candida, Aspergillus, and Histoplasma. Parasite: An organism that lives on a host species to obtain food. Examples: Whipworm, tapeworm, amoeba.

Protozoa

Protozoa is a single-celled animal with a membrane nucleus (eukaryotic), which can be visible to the naked eye. Flagella and cilia make them motile for hunting food. Examples: Amoeba, paramecia, and trypanosomes.

TB infection

The tests that identify tuberculosis infection (TB) are a positive Mantoux skin test or QFT-G blood test. Both must be confirmed by chest x-ray and sputum culture. 10% of exposed persons with positive Mantoux tests develop active TB infection. Your employer offers you prophylaxis with Isoniazid (INH) if you are exposed to an active TB case.

To perform the two-step Mantoux skin test:
- Week 1: The CMA injects 0.1 ml of 5 units tuberculin intradermally in the patient's forearm
- 2 or 3 days later: The patient returns to have the test read. A negative test has no redness or swelling
- Week 2 or 3: The CMA repeats the test again to prevent identification of a booster reaction as a positive TB result

Patients with AIDS, lupus, renal failure, or kidney transplant have false-negative reactions to Mantoux. The patient who received BCG vaccine against TB will have a false-positive reaction. Ask the registered nurse to perform the QFT-G blood test for these patients, instead of Mantoux.

12 leads of an EKG

An EKG lead is the wire and electrode that connects the patient to the electrocardiograph machine (also abbreviated ECG). A standard 12-lead EKG actually has only 10 wires and electrodes, which record 12 electrical vectors:

Unipolar Leads:
- Augmented Vector Right (AVR) [right atrial view]
- Augmented Vector Left (AVL) [lateral view]
- Augmented Vector Foot (AVF) [inferior view]
- Precordial chest lead V1 [anterior view]
- Precordial chest lead V2 [anterior view]
- Precordial chest lead V3 [septal view]
- Precordial chest lead V4 [septal view]
- Precordial chest lead V5 [lateral view]
- Precordial chest lead V6 [lateral view]

Bipolar Leads:
- Limb lead I [lateral view]
- Limb lead II [inferior view]
- Limb lead III [inferior view]

Rarely, a cardiologist who suspects damage to the rear wall of the heart that is not evident on a 12-lead will ask for V8 and V9 on the patient's back.

Visual acuity testing

Distance vision
Tape a line on the floor exactly 20 feet from a well-lit eye chart.
- Place the Snellen chart at the patient's eye level
- Perform the test first with the patient's glasses or contact lenses in place
- Position your patient at the floor line
- Give your patient an eye pad or paper cup
- Tell your patient to keep both eyes open, but to cover the right eye with the pad or cup
- Stand beside the eye chart and point to the letters
- Ask your patient to read the letters aloud, line by line, from the top down
- The line on which a patient makes an error is his/her visual acuity for distance
- Record the reading beside the line in the patient's chart (e.g., 20/50)
- The top number is the distance the patient stands from the chart, 20 feet
- The bottom number indicates the distance from which a person with normal vision could read the same line
- For example, a patient with 20/40 vision can read the line 20 feet away that a person with normal sight can see clearly from 40 feet away
- Repeat with the left eye
- Tell the patient to remove his/her glasses or contact lenses

- Provide a sink, soap, towel, lens case and saline, if the patient with contacts requires them
- Repeat the test without glasses or contact lenses

Near vision

Repeat the test with a Jaeger card held 14 inches from the patient's face.

Normal visual acuity

(VA) is 20/20, meaning the patient can read the eighth line down on a Snellen eye chart from a distance of 20 feet away.

The refractive errors are:
- *Myopia*: The patient sees nearby objects clearly but objects in the distance are blurry because the eye is too long. The patient can read the Jaeger card but not the Snellen wall chart, and requires glasses for driving and distance vision
- *Presbyopia*: Around age 45, the aging patient's lenses become inelastic and his/her eyes do not focus well on nearby objects. The patient can see the Snellen wall chart well, but not the Jaeger card, and requires reading glasses
- *Hyperopia*: The eye may be too small or the focusing power too weak, so the patient is unable to see objects nearby (far-sighted). The patient can read the Snellen chart, but not the Jaeger card, and requires glasses
- *Astigmatism*: The patient's cornea and/or lens are not smooth; they have irregular curvatures, with flat and steep

sections that blur sections of the visual field

Basic audiology testing

Audiology testing measures the ability of the patient's inner ear to hear sounds through varying degrees of loudness (intensity) and vibration speed (tone). The audiometer measures intensity in decibels (dB) and tone in Hertz (Hz or cycles per second).
- A whisper is 20 Hz and 20 dB
- Prolonged sounds louder than 85 dB cause hearing loss
- A loud concert is 100 dB
- The bass plays at 50 Hz, and the high violin plays at 10,000 Hz
- Normal hearing range is 20 Hz to 20,000 Hz
- Speech ranges from 500 to 3,000 Hz

If an adult cannot hear a ticking watch or a whisper, he/she needs an audiology test, which takes about 10 minutes.
- The doctor taps a tuning fork and holds it on the sides of the patient's head to find if he/she can hear sound conducted through air
- The doctor taps the tuning fork and holds it behind the patient's ear on the mastoid bone to find if he/she can hear sound conducted by vibration through bone
- The CMA places earphones on the patient and connects them to the audiometer

- The CMA attaches a bone oscillator to the patient's mastoid bones
- The CMA runs pure tones through one earpiece at a time, and controls the intensity
- The patient either raises one hand or presses a button when he/she hears a tone
- The CMA records on a graph the minimum intensity the patient needs to hear each tone
- The patient should be able to hear 250 Hz to 8,000 Hz at 25 dB or lower
- If he/she cannot hear below 25 dB, then there is hearing loss

PFTs

Pulmonary function tests (PFTs) measure how much air the patient's lungs can hold, how fast air can be moved in and out of the patient's lungs, and how well the lungs retain oxygen and discard carbon dioxide. Use an interpretation table, because PFT varies by age, body mass, gender, and race.

- Seat the patient
- Place a clip over his/her nose
- The patient inhales to full capacity and exhales completely into a spirometer for 6 seconds
- Repeat twice and take the best reading out of three, measured in liters

Tidal Volume (TV) is one normal inhalation and exhalation. Inspiratory Reserve Volume (IRV) is the most volume the patient can inhale after a complete breath. Expiratory Reserve Volume (ERV) is the most volume a patient can exhale forcefully after one normal exhalation. Residual Volume (RV) is the amount of air remaining in the lungs after the patient exhales forcefully. Minute volume is the air inhaled and exhaled in one minute of normal breathing. Vital capacity is TV + IRV + ERV.
Total lung capacity is TV + IRV + ERV + RV.

Pulse rate varies by age:

Normal Resting Pulse Rate	Age
60—100 beats per minute	Adult
80—100 beats per minute	Child
100 beats per minute	Toddler
100—140 beats per minute	Infant under one year
up to 150 beats per minute	Newborn (neonate)

If you cannot feel a distal pulse in your patient's limbs, find the apical pulse in the chest. Count to the 5th rib space in the middle of the left side of the chest or midclavicular line. If the apical pulse is regular, count for 30 seconds and record the reading. If the apical pulse is irregular, count for a full minute and record the reading.

Report an irregular pulse to the doctor to evaluate for possible pulse deficit. A pulse deficit occurs when the radial pulse in the wrist is slower than the apical pulse in the chest. A pulse deficit can indicate your patient has weak heart contractions, which fail to transmit beats to the arterial system.

The radial pulse is palpated at the wrist, under the thumb. When taking a pulse, you should use the pads of your index finger and middle finger. Your thumb has a pulse beat of it's own, which may interfere with feeling the patient's pulse.

Pulse

The pulse is a surge of blood through an artery that occurs when the heart contracts (systole).

The key pulse points are:
- Apical over the heart
- Brachial in the elbow bend (for children under 1 year)
- Carotid in the neck (for unconscious patients)
- Dorsalis pedis on top of the foot
- Facial on the jaw under the mouth
- Femoral in the thigh
- Popliteal on the back of the knee
- Posterior tibial on the back of the ankle
- *Quest 2* Radial on the wrist below the thumb (most common in patients older than 1 year)
- Temporal on the temple
- Ulnar on the wrist below the little finger

Use direct pressure on the pulse point nearest a cut to control bleeding. Evaluate the extremities for healthy circulation by palpating the distal pulses. The doctor rubs the carotid arteries on both sides of the patient's neck as vagus nerve stimulation (VNS) therapy to decrease pulse rate in tachycardia.

Patient's vital signs

Stable vital signs in the normal range indicate good health (homeostasis). Ill or injured patients have vital signs outside the normal range. The severity of the illness or injury often is indicated by the variability of vital sign measurements. Look for variations from previous visits. Wide variations mean the patient is unstable; check the vital signs every 5 minutes. In stable patients, check the vital signs every 15 minutes.

Tachycardia

Tachycardia is a pulse rate over 100 beats per minute, which may be caused by: Anxiety; fear; stress; pneumonia; anemia; low blood pressure; dehydration; hyperthyroidism; and heart conditions.

Bradycardia

Bradycardia is a resting heart rate less than 60 beats per minute, which may be caused by: Heart attack (MI); hypothermia; heat exhaustion; obstructive jaundice; skull fracture; malnutrition; hypothyroidism; and many adverse drug reactions. Olympic athletes may have bradycardia because their hearts are extremely efficient.

Safe medical imaging

Medical Imaging includes:
- X-rays (radiographs)
- CAT (computerized axial tomography)
- MRI (magnetic resonance imaging)
- Ultrasound; and contrast and barium studies

Check the patient's allergy alerts recorded in the chart, particularly for latex and contrast dye, and alert the radiology technologist (RT) if necessary.

- If your patient may be pregnant, perform a pregnancy test before imaging and inform the patient and RT if it is positive
- Tell your patient to wear loose, comfortable clothing
- Explain that he/she may need to don a gown because metal snaps, zippers, buttons and fasteners interfere with imaging
- Dentures, hearing aids, eyeglasses, hairpins, credit cards, watches, jewelry, and keys must be placed in the locker provided or left with an attendant because they interfere with imaging
- Metal jewelry worn in body piercings and new tattoos are dangerous because they heat up during MRI scans
- Your patient must remove the jewelry and may need to wait until the dye becomes safe before imaging
- Contact the RT for specific directions that vary by test, and relay them to your patient (e.g., fast 8 hours; drink a liter of water; take a laxative and enema the night before)

Preparing and administering medications

Controlled substances

Controlled substances are categorized under the Controlled Substances Act of 1970. There are five groups of controlled substances, numbered Schedule I to Schedule V.

- Schedule I substances have a high potential for abuse and dependence and have NO accepted medical use in the United States. These drugs are not considered safe to use even under medical supervision. Schedule I substances are for research and instructional purposes only. Schedule I drugs include Ecstasy, China White, and LSD
- Schedule II substances have a high potential for abuse, but have an accepted medical use. Use is severely restricted because severe psychological and/or physical dependence may develop. Schedule II drugs include Amytal, PCP, Ritalin, and Dexedrine
- Schedule III substances have less potential for abuse than Schedule I and II substances, and have an accepted medical use in the United States. Abuse of these substances may lead to moderate or low physical dependence and/or high psychological dependence. Schedule III drugs include anabolic steroids for body building, like Winstrol, and amobarbital/ephedrine capsules
- Schedule IV drugs have a low potential for abuse compared to substances in Schedule III. Schedule IV substances have an accepted medical use in the United States. Abuse of substances in this category may lead to limited physical

and/or psychological dependence. Examples of Schedule IV drugs are Xanax, Librium, Valium, and the date rape drug Rohypnol
- Schedule V substances have a low potential for abuse compared to Schedule IV drugs. Schedule V substances have an accepted medical use in the United States. Abuse of Schedule V drugs may lead to limited physical and/or psychological dependence compared to Schedule IV substances. Examples of Schedule V drugs are Robitussin A-C, Lomotil, Thymergix, and Pediacof

Common drug manuals for the medical office are:
- The American Drug Index, Compendium of Pharmaceuticals and Specialties
- Lippincott's Nursing Drug Guide and Stoklosa's Pharmaceutical Calculations
- The definitive on-line drug reference is the The United States Pharmacopeia–National Formulary (USP–NF) at http://www.usp.org/USPNF/
- When in doubt about a drug, always contact a pharmacist

Side-effect

Side effect is an unwanted effect of a therapeutic dose of a drug. A side-effect may or may not cause the patient harm. An example is drowsiness for cold medications.

AE

Adverse event (AE) is a minor side-effect that may or may not be expected. For example, a patient may develop indigestion after using Aspirin for a headache.

SE

Sentinel event (SE) is an unexpected outcome causing serious physical or psychological harm, or even death. For example, a child may develop brain damage from Reyes Syndrome after taking Aspirin for influenza.

Substance abuse

Substance abuse is excessive use of any substance, but usually drugs or alcohol, which impairs or distresses a patient for 12 months or more. Substance abuse is characterized by failure at school, work, or home due to frequent absences, neglect, or bizarre behavior. Substance abuse produces legal problems, such as arrests for disorderly conduct or driving while impaired. The abuser continues to crave the substance despite its physical hazards and social problems.

Drug administration

The route of administration is the manner by which a drug is introduced into the body. The routes of administration are:
- Enteral (oral, rectal, or by feeding tube)
- Topical (on the skin, in the eyes or nose, vaginal, or inhaled)
- Parenteral (IV, subcutaneous, intramuscular, intracardiac,

intraosseous, intradermal, intrathecal, intraperitoneal, transdermal, transmucosal, intravitreal, and epidural)

The route of administration affects the way the medication is taken up, distributed, and eliminated. The effect of a medication is local or systemic. There are many variations on these three basic routes of administration. The FDA acknowledges 111 different routes of administration. When deciding on the route of administration, the doctor and pharmacist consider:

- How fast the patient requires the drug
- How effective it will be by a given route
- The likelihood of toxicity
- The discomfort it will cause
- How likely the patient is to comply with the route
- How likely the route is to play into the patient's addictive habits

Calculating drug dosage

The CMA must weigh the patient accurately because the registered nurse (RN) usually calculates drug dosage by milligrams of medication per kilogram of patient's body weight. For example, if the drug reference manual states the general dosage is 20 mg/kg and the child patient weighs 25 kg (55 lbs), then the patient receives 500 mg.

However, some drugs have a maximum dosage that must not be exceeded within 24 hours, regardless of the patient's weight. Divide the maximum dosage by the general dosage to find out if a child gets an adult dose. For example, the maximum dose is 600 mg and the general dosage is 20 mg/kg. The child who weighs 31 kg (68 lbs) gets an adult dose but the child who weighs 25 kg (55 lbs) gets a pediatric dose.

Sometimes the doctor's prescription is different from the available dosage. For example, the pharmacist has 250 mg capsules of ampicillin in stock but the doctor's prescription calls for a dose of 500 mg. divide the required dose by the available dose. This patient gets two 250 mg. capsules to equal 500 mg.

Injections

Subcutaneous injection
Deliver the drug under the skin with a ½ inch, 24 or 25 gauge needle held at a 45° angle to reach the fat. Choose the upper arm, abdomen, thigh or lower back as the site. The maximum amount of SubQ medication is 0.5 ml. An example is insulin for a patient with diabetes.

Intramuscular injection
Deliver the drug into the muscle with a 1 inch long, 20 gauge needle held at a 90° angle perpendicular to the muscle, to reach the deep tissue. For obese patients, use a 2 inch needle. Choose the vastus lateralis (thigh), ventrogluteal (hip), deltoid (upper arm), or dorsogluteal (buttocks) as the site. The maximum amount of IM medication is 5 ml. An example is Vitamin B12 for a patient with pernicious anemia.

Intravenous injection

Deliver the drug into a vein of the arm, hand, leg, foot, scalp or neck with an Angiocath, butterfly, or InSyte Autoguard needle. Use a size from 14 gauge to 26 gauge, depending on the fluid and the patient. The nurse sets the drip rate per minute by adjusting the clamp and monitoring the drip chamber. An example is Zolendronate that is given yearly to prevent bone fractures for individuals with osteoporosis.

Two less frequently used forms of injection are:
- Intradermal (into the skin) for Mantoux TB test
- Intraosseus access (IO) into the sternum, which an ambulance team uses for an emergency case

Drug storage

Correct storage maintains a drug's efficacy and safety. Store most drugs at room temperature (22°C up to 25°C); protect drugs from insects, dust, light and humidity. Patients and visitors should not be able to see your automated dispensing cabinet or drug cupboard. Keep all drugs out of the reach of children, known drug addicts, and patients who may be suicidal. Some biologicals, especially ointments, hormones and vaccines, require refrigeration.

Improper storage causes the drug to degrade before its expiration date. Most drugs last 2 to 5 years from their date of manufacture, providing they are kept in ideal conditions. However, some specialty preparations, such as eye drops, may only last a few hours, days or weeks.

Controlled drugs

Controlled drugs are supervised by the Drug Enforcement Administration (DEA) and include human anesthetics, analgesics, sedatives, and drugs used to euthanize animals. Controlled drugs must be double locked in a wall cabinet and the key must not be kept nearby, record use in a log. When the drug expires or the bottle is empty, return the log and bottle to Pharmacy.

Immunization schedule

Travelers to exotic locations and healthcare workers need additional vaccines. Pregnant women, HIV patients, diabetics, alcoholics, COPD, liver, kidney and spleen disease patients have different needs and do not fit this schedule.

2010 CDC vaccination schedule 0 – 6 years

Hepatitis B	Birth the second at 1 to 2 months and the third at 6 to 18 months. If high risk, the shot should be given within 12 hours of birth, at age 1-2 months followed by the third shot at 6 months.
Rotavirus	2, 4 and 6 months
Diphtheria, Tetanus and Pertussis (DTP)	2, 4 and 6 months, 15 to 18 months and 4 to 6 years
Haemophilus influenzae Type B	2, 4 and 6 months, and at 12 to 15 months
Pneumococcus	2 and 4 and 6 months, and at 12 to 15 months
Inactivated Polio	2 and 4 months, 6 to 18 months, and a booster at 4 to 6 years
Influenza	Yearly
Measles, Mumps, Rubella	12 to 15months and 4 to 6 years
Hepatitis A	Two doses from 12 months to 2 years at least 6 months apart
Meningococcal	MCV 2 to 6 years only if high risk
Varicella (chickenpox)	12-15 months followed by a second dose at 4-6 years

CDC vaccination schedule for 2010 for 7 to 18 years

Hepatitis B	Catch-up 7 to 18
Diphtheria, Tetanus and Pertussis (Tdap)	Regular 11-12 years; catch-up 13 to 18
Human Papilloma Virus (HPV)	No younger than 9; regular three doses 11 to 12 (with the third dose at least 24 weeks after the first dose); catch-up 13 to 18
Pneumococcus	High risk 7 to 18
Inactivated Polio	Catch-up 7 to 18
Influenza	Yearly
Measles, Mumps, Rubella & Varicella	Catch-up 7 to 18
Hepatitis A	High risk 7 to 18
Meningococcal	High risk 7 to 10; regular 11 to 12; catch-up 13 to 18

CDC vaccination schedule for adults

Hepatitis B	High risk individuals should be given 3 doses over a 4 month period
Diphtheria, Tetanus and Pertussis	Tdap 19 to 64 who have not previously received Tdap. Td booster every 10 years thereafter
Human Papilloma Virus	Females only 19 to 26 three doses if not previously infected with HPV
Pneumococcus (PPSV)	If medically indicated, one or two doses 19 to 64; one dose over 65
Influenza	Yearly
Measles, Mumps, Rubella &	For those C born after 1957 should receive 2 doses 4 weeks apart.
Varicella (chickenpox)	Adults without evidence of immunity should receive 2 doses 4-8 weeks apart
Herpes Zoster	One dose over age 60 even if prior case of zoster
Hepatitis A	Two doses over age 19 if high risk
Meningococcal	One or more doses between 19 and old age if high risk

- 97 -

Store vaccines

The following rules apply for routine vaccines, such as flu, DTaP, Hib, HepB, PCV7, PPV23, and EIPV: Protect vaccines from light.

- Never store a vaccine on the refrigerator door
- Always keep open vials of vaccine on a tray in the main refrigerator compartment
- Keep a liquid or mercury thermometer on the same shelf as the vaccine tray
- Check and record the thermometer reading twice per day, when your shift starts and before you leave, and record it in a log
- The refrigerator ideally should be 40ºF (5ºC), but must be 36ºF to 46ºF (2ºC to 8ºC)
- Varicella and MMR must be frozen, ideally at 0ºF, but the freezer must be 5ºF or colder (-15ºC to -20ºC)
- Use a plug guard on the refrigerator and post a sign on it that reads "Biologicals" with a biohazard sign
- NEVER store food or specimens in the same refrigerator as vaccines
- Rotate stock weekly, so the oldest vaccine is used first
- A vaccine marked only with month and year is viable until the last day of the month
- Never use expired vaccine
- Never pre-draw vaccine or leave it out of the refrigerator between uses
- During transport, keep refrigerated vaccines in an insulated container on a cold gel pack, and use dry ice for frozen vaccines
- Report all accidents to the Safety Officer and do not use compromised vaccine

If you encounter an unusual vaccine, read the product insert, refer to The Red Book if the insert is missing, or phone the manufacturer.

Standard crash cart

A standard crash cart contains a green oxygen tank, masks, airways, a defibrillator, and resuscitation drugs. One crash cart should be available per floor; remember where it is located. In an emergency, here are the CMA's duties:

- Tell the receptionist to call an ambulance (911) and notify the doctor, or do so yourself if there is no receptionist
- Place the patient in recovery position (side-lying) while you obtain the crash cart
- Reposition the patient in the Trendelenburg position, lying on the back with feet raised above chest level
- Apply direct pressure to a wound to stop bleeding, if necessary
- Position the oxygen mask over the patient's nose, with tubing to the side. Fasten the mask firmly. Administer oxygen immediately, from 2 and 4 liters per minute. If the patient is still conscious, explain that he/she must breathe through the nose with the mouth closed
- Try to calm and comfort the patient. Cover the patient with

a blanket to help prevent shock. Screen the patient from public view
- Prepare to start CPR, if necessary
- The doctor or registered nurse intubates the unconscious patient and administers resuscitation drugs, assist as required
- If there is no receptionist, wait at the door to guide the ambulance attendants to the patient

Emergencies

AED

An automated external defibrillator (AED) can revive a person who is in cardiac arrest, providing it is applied within four minutes and damage is not extensive.

- Continue CPR until the unit is charged
- You must be on a flat, dry surface
- Connect the electrodes of the AED to the patient, as illustrated on the unit
- Press the "analyze" button first for a readout, to ensure the unit is ready and electroshock is appropriate
- Announce, "Stay clear of the patient"
- Restart CPR if defibrillation is contraindicated
- The unit indicates by tone or light that it is ready to shock the patient

- The AED display shows when defibrillation occurs
- Test the pulse after the third shock
- If there is a pulse, check the airway, breathing circulation and move the patient into recovery position
- If there is no pulse, perform CPR for one minute before rechecking the pulse
- If there is still no pulse, defibrillate again
- Press the analysis button
- Nine defibrillations can be performed in total
- The unit indicates when to stop defibrillation

Triage

Triage means dividing casualties into one of three groups: immediate, delayed, or nontransport. The triage officer commands, and should be the most qualified individual, regardless of rank and seniority. Primary triage is conducted at the scene of the incident. The triage group sort's patients according to the severity of their injuries with a color coding system:

- A red tag indicates a first priority patient
- A yellow tag indicates a second priority patient
- A green tag indicates a delayed priority patient
- Colored ribbon, tape, or labels are also appropriate

Secondary triage is conducted in the treatment area to prioritize medical care and transportation to hospital. The treatment group arranges the medical care for patients after they have been triaged. The supply group obtains necessary resources and distributes these as needed. Your transportation officer contacts the receiving hospital about the incoming casualties. The staging group directs incoming ambulances. The extrication group frees trapped patients.

Minimal documentation is required for triage because treatment is top priority. Complete documentation after attending to the casualties.

START system

START is a triage system used at multi-casualty incidents. The acronym stands for Simple Triage And Rapid Treatment. START assesses patients using three parameters: Respiration, perfusion, and mentation. These parameters spell RPM. The assessment of a patient using START takes no more than 30 seconds. Patients are triaged using START according to:

- The patient's ability to walk away from the incident site
- Whether respiratory rate is under or over 30 respirations per minute
- Whether capillary refill is over or under 2 seconds and/or whether the patient has a radial pulse
- Whether the patient is able to follow basic commands

Ensure your own safety, the safety of the general public, and the safety of the patient, in that order. Don appropriate personal protective equipment (PPE) before approaching a contaminated patient. Identifying a hazardous substance should not take precedence over the health and safety of your patient. Fire department officials or a Haz-Mat team are better able to identify the hazard. CMAs are not generally responsible for securing or controlling the scene of the emergency; that is a police function.

Emergency preparedness information

To access the CDC's free tools for emergency preparedness visit:
- http://emergency.cdc.gov/pre paredness/.

Your Safety Officer and your facility's Incident Management System (IMS) must ensure that you have proper emergency training and equipment.

CMAs must recertify in CPR with the American Red Cross or the American Heart Association every two years at the Healthcare Provider Level. All staff must attend emergency preparedness training. This includes fire, natural disasters, severe weather, and CBRN (chemical, biological, radiation, and nuclear training against terrorism). The role of each person in the medical office during an emergency must be clearly identified in the job description. For example:
- The front desk receptionist phones EMS, notifies the doctor, directs traffic, and reschedules patients
- The CMA obtains the crash cart, provides first aid, and assists the doctor with life support
- The nurse administers drugs, first aid, and contacts the

patient's next-of-kin and physician

- The doctor leads two-person CPR and administers resuscitation drugs
- You must rehearse and cross-train
- Long-term inpatients and outpatients who are on the premises for extended periods (e.g. dialysis) and are capable of understanding and participating are required to have evacuation training
- Good Samaritan Act and duty of care

Good Samaritan Act

There are two kinds of Good Samaritan Acts:

- A first aider who provides unpaid assistance to the injured in an emergency and acts as "a reasonable man" up to his/her level of training is protected by state law from unfair prosecution for death, disability, or disfigurement. A judge would dismiss assault and battery charges. A Good Samaritan Act is not a duty to assist law, except in Vermont and Minnesota. Nevada and California may adopt a duty to assist clause
- A living donor who offers a non-directed donation of an organ to the transplant center is a Good Samaritan. The following organs can be donated by a living donor: kidneys; liver lobes; lung lobes; pancreas segments; and small bowel segments.

- Non-direct donors do not have anyone particular in mind that they would like to receive their donated organ. The donation is usually anonymous and the Good Samaritan is blameless for complications the recipient suffers

Duty of care

The CMA must act as "a reasonable man" and meet the standard of care to avoid negligence charges. This means being watchful, attentive, cautious, and prudent at work.

Treatment for bleeding

When direct pressure on an injury does not stop bleeding, exert indirect pressure with the flats of your fingers or thumb on the nearest pulse (pressure point).

- Compressing the artery against a bone where they are both close to the skin surface usually stops bleeding
- If the fingers are insufficient, use the heel of your hand
- Indirect pressure results in inadequate blood flow to an area and can cause tissue damage from ischemia
- Use indirect pressure cautiously
- Applying pressure to the carotid artery can cause cardiac arrest or stroke
- The brachial artery is the pressure point to control bleeding in the forearm
- The femoral artery is the pressure point to control bleeding from the leg

- The subclavian artery controls upper chest and neck bleeding
- The temporal artery and facial artery control bleeding in the face and neck

Only use a tourniquet to control bleeding when all other methods have failed, and only on the extremities, not the trunk or head.
- Write the letters TK and the time you applied the tourniquet on the patient's forehead
- Release the tourniquet every 5 minutes to allow circulation
- The patient may lose the limb due to ischemia

Natural disaster

When a natural disaster strikes a community, the Multi-Agency Coordination System (MACS) responds. EMS (police, fire department, and ambulance), Red Cross, and military Search and Rescue teams conduct rescue efforts. Healthcare facilities and community agencies, such as Public Health, the CDC, and community care nurses, are second-line responders. Mass casualties require the assistance of private doctors and allied health personnel, so you may be seconded to help away from your usual post. Public buildings, such as schools, sports arenas and churches, are used as shelters. Extra medical supplies, food, clean water, and morgues are secured by deputies in case of looting. U.S. states and Canadian provinces follow the Standardized Emergency Management System (SEMS) for natural disaster preparedness,

mitigation, response and recovery. Your facility's manager helps to set up the Incident Command System (ICS) for the healthcare facility. The Administrator On-call liaises with community leaders and designates a spokesperson for the healthcare facility.

First aid

Burn treatment

The types of burns are thermal, chemical, electrical, radiation, and mechanical.
- A first degree (superficial) burn is damage to the epidermis with reddening and moderate pain
- A second degree (partial-thickness) burn involves the epidermis and dermis with reddening, blistering, and severe pain
- A third degree (full-thickness) burn extends through the epidermis, dermis, and deep tissues, such as muscle and bone
- It may be leathery and white or charred, and is not painful where nerves are destroyed
- A respiratory tract burn (inhalation injury) produces sooty nasal hairs, nostrils, or lips and a hoarse voice or stridorous breathing

To begin treatment for a first- or second- degree burn, remove your patient from the burning agent.

- Gently remove clothing and jewelry from the affected area, provided they are not sticking, because burns swell
- If there is chemical powder, brush it from the patient with cardboard so it does not react with water
- Flush the burn with cool water for 20 minutes
- If skin is sloughing, immerse the burn in cold water
- Do not use ice
- If you cannot flush or immerse the burn, wrap it in clean cloth soaked in cool water
- Do not apply butter
- After the burn has cooled, the wound should be loosely covered with sterile gauze
- An over the counter pain reliever such as ibuprofen or acetaminophen should be given
- For major burns, call 911 immediately
- Your patient needs an antibacterial silver bandage, an analgesic, and possibly IV fluid replacement therapy

Rule of nines

You will hear the Rule of Nines when transcribing:
- In an adult, each part of the body contributes the following percentage to the entire body surface area: Perineum, 1%; each leg, 18%; each arm, 9%; chest and abdomen, 18%; back and buttocks, 18%; and head, 9%
- In a child, each part of the body contributes the following percentage to the entire body surface area: Each leg, 16%; each arm, 9%; chest and abdomen, 18%; back and buttocks, 18%; and head, 14%
- In an infant, each part of the body contributes the following percentage to the entire body surface area: Each leg, 14%; each arm, 9%; chest and abdomen, 18%, back and buttocks, 18%, and head, 18%. The palm of the hand and groin are each 1% of the entire body surface

The ER doctor uses the Rule of Nines to determine when to give fluid resuscitation (20—25%) and when to transfer the patient to the Burn Unit. Burns to the face and palms are usually critical.

Choking victim

If your patient is reclined, anesthetized, eating, or has a slippery objects in the mouth, a foreign body airway obstruction (FBAO) may occur.
- The universal distress signal for FBAO is clutching of the throat with both hands
- If the patient does this, suspend treatment immediately
- A choking patient cannot speak
- Breathing is difficult or absent
- The mouth may be blue (cyanotic)
- Ask the patient to sit up and cough
- If he/she cannot force out the foreign body independently, call for help

- 103 -

- Perform the Heimlich maneuver to open the blocked airway
- If the patient is conscious, stand behind him/her
- Wrap your arms around the patient's abdomen
- Make one hand into a fist; grasp the other hand firmly over it
- Deliver a series of swift subdiaphragmatic thrusts, until the airway is clear or the patient falls unconscious
- The patient needs follow-up medical treatment in case the airway was damaged

Abdominal thrusts procedure

If a patient with foreign body airway obstruction (FBAO) becomes unconscious during the standing Heimlich maneuver, phone Emergency Medical Services (EMS) immediately. Brain death occurs in 4 to 6 minutes.

- Place the patient on his/her back
- Don gloves
- Lift the tongue and jaw and sweep the mouth with your fingers to remove the foreign body
- Open the airway by tilting the head, lifting the chin, pinching the nose
- Insert a resuscitation mask into the mouth
- Blow two slow breaths into the airway
- Repositioning of the head may be required
- If the airway remains obstructed, then landmark the xiphoid process
- Straddle the patient's thighs

- Position the heels of both hands just below the xiphoid notch at the base of the sternum
- One hand is on top of the other
- Apply 5 abdominal thrusts, pressing toward the diaphragm
- Continue thrusting until the airway is unblocked or EMS arrives to take over

Single-rescuer CPR

Call Emergency Medical Services (911) before beginning cardiopulmonary resuscitation (CPR). Only perform CPR on a patient with cardiac arrest, who is unresponsive, with no pulse or breathing.

- Don gloves, if possible
- Place the patient supine on the floor
- Look, listen, and feel for the patient's breathing
- If there is none, open the patient's airway by inclining the head back and raising the chin
- Place a resuscitation mouthpiece into the patient's mouth
- Pinch the nose closed
- Inflate the lungs with two breaths
- Observe the chest's rise and fall
- Check the carotid pulse for about 15 seconds
- If no pulse is present, kneel beside the patient
- Landmark the xiphoid process at the end of the sternum (breastbone), where the ribs meet
- Place your palms over the breastbone

- 104 -

- Compress 30 times, followed by two breaths
- After four cycles, check the carotid pulse again
- Continue until the patient breathes or you are relieved by a rescuer with higher training
- Discard the mouthpiece
- Document CPR in the patient's chart

Diabetic coma vs. diabetic shock

Diabetic coma results from prolonged high blood sugar (hyperglycemia) caused by too much sugar or carbohydrates and not enough insulin; initially, the patient's mental status alters.

- He/she is confused, thirsty, and exhibits drunken behavior
- The patient urinates frequently and may vomit
- He/she complains of nausea and abdominal pain
- The skin is flushed and dry
- The patient snores when he/she eventually sinks into coma
- Ketones will be present in the urine, the blood sugar level will be elevated and the patient's breath may have a fruity odor
- Stop the procedure
- The patient will require insulin
- Fluid replacement is required. Inform the doctor

Diabetic shock is also known as insulin shock and results from sudden low blood sugar (hypoglycemia, glucose less than 70 mg/dl) through fasting, overexertion, alcohol ingestion, stress, or drug reactions.

- The patient displays nervousness, irritability, shaking, cold sweats, and complains of hunger
- Loss of consciousness follows
- Stop the procedure
- The rule of 15 should be followed where 15 grams of carbohydrate is given then the blood glucose can be rechecked in 15 minutes
- Give 4 ounces of orange juice, or a glucose drink, or 3-4 glucose tablets, or 6-8 Lifesavers candies immediately
- A delay may cause your patient to become unresponsive and require glucagon injections, or hospital treatment for acidosis
- If the blood glucose is still low after 15 minutes, the procedure should be repeated

Fractures

A fracture is a break or disruption in the integrity of a bone that occurs when force or weight are applied to the bone, which exceed the bone's ability to remain structurally intact. Fractures occur from direct or indirect trauma, or because of diseases (e.g., cancer and osteoporosis) and congenital states such as contractures. Fractures are frequently associated with adjacent soft tissue injuries. Modern fractures are classified as either open or closed.

Older fracture classifications still used in transcriptions include:
- Simple (skin intact, no bone contact with air); compound (bone protrudes through skin)
- Comminuted (splintered)

- 105 -

- Compacted (bone ends are jammed together)
- Spiral (twisted, as in a skiing accident)
- Compression (where the patient loses height because the spine fuses)
- Oblique (diagonal to the axis); transverse (right angled to the axis)
- Linear (parallel to the axis)
- Incomplete (bone is still joined at some points)
- Complete (bone fragments are completely separated)
- Greenstick (twisted immature bones)

Fracture treatment
Observe the patient for:
- Angulation, bones shifted out of their normal position
- Deformity or swelling
- Guarding, holding the injured part or favoring it
- Inability to use the part
- Paradoxical breathing movements
- Rotation, a bone fragment turned around its central axis

The goals of the CMA are to:
- Immobilize the area with bandages or splints to prevent further injury and pain, the mechanism of injury
- Call EMS for transportation to the nearest Emergency Room for x-ray

Look for associated injuries, such as flail chest and pneumothorax.
- If it is an open fracture, apply a dressing to control bleeding, prevent further contamination, and minimize psychogenic shock because the patient does not have to look at the injury
- Burns that cause fractures are critical
- Fractures or dislocations involving the vertebral column can cause spinal cord injuries and paralysis so do not move the patient
- Clear yellow cerebrospinal fluid or blood leaking from the ear, nose, or eyes indicates a skull fracture

Medications for ingested poison

Syrup of ipecac induces vomiting. Activated charcoal pills or slurry absorb poison. Your choice depends on the type of poison the patient ingested:
- If it burned the esophagus on the way down (e.g., petroleum distillates or lye), then it will burn on the way up. Therefore, dilute the corrosive poison with 2 cups of water or milk. Do not induce vomiting
- If the patient ingested cyanide, a medication, or a non-corrosive substance AND is completely conscious, then induce vomiting with ipecac or salt water. However, do not give syrup of ipecac if the patient ingested more than 400 mg/kg of ibuprofen or mefenamic acid. Never make a semi-conscious or unconscious patient vomit. You may give water and multiple doses of charcoal (charcoal slurry) after

the patient stops vomiting to dilute and absorb the residue

- When the doctor arrives, assist him/her with gastric lavage and neutralizing the ingested substance, if required. Depending on the pH, the doctor may neutralize a base with vinegar or lemon juice, or neutralize an acid with baking soda

Epilepsy

Epilepsy is an electric storm in the brain from uncontrolled, synchronized firing of neurons. Epilepsy can be acquired from head injury or innate, from neural membranes abnormally permeable to sodium and potassium. Anticonvulsants like Tegretol, phenobarb and Dilantin control epilepsy.

Absence

An absence is a generalized seizure, formerly called petit mal, with no specific focus in the brain. The patient stares, lip smacks, and blinks for a few seconds. Absences begin and end without warning and are difficult to discern because there is no after-effect. However, a 3 Hz spike and wave discharges result on an EEG. Absence seizures interfere with learning. The patient is unaware of what occurred during the seizure. Youths 7—19 are prone to seizures from flashing strobe lights at discos and flickering TV patterns. A famous case is the December 1997 Pokémon episode that sent 700 children to hospital; 500 had confirmed seizures.

Tonic-clonic seizure

Tonic-clonic seizure (grand mal) is a convulsion involving the entire brain. An aura may precede the seizure (smell, lights, or other warning symptom). Muscles contract during tonic phase, breathing is irregular, and skin is blue tinged from lack of oxygen (cyanosis). The patient loses bladder control. In clonic phase, limbs jerk from quick muscle contraction and relaxation. After the seizure, the patient is limp, regains consciousness gradually, and is confused. Recovery takes hours.

Stroke

Signs and symptoms of stroke (cerebrovascular accident or CVA) include:

- Disruptions in vision
- Trouble speaking or expressing thoughts; headache
- Weakness affecting one side of the body
- Difficulty walking
- Numbness or tingling on one side of the body

Loss of consciousness is rare. The patient may be having a transient ischemic attack (TIA or mini-stroke), which is a warning of an impending stroke.

- Give the patient 2 Aspirins and call EMS (911)
- Place the patient in recovery position with the affected side down, the head slightly elevated, and cover him/her with a blanket
- Bring the crash cart

- Paramedics will ask the patient to smile, to extend the arms for 10 seconds with the eyes closed, and to repeat a phrase
- The base hospital doctor may order the paramedics to administer dipyridamole (Persantine), clopidogrel (Plavix), or ticlopidine (Ticlid)
- Approximately 33% of patients who experience a transient ischemic attack will have recurrent attacks

Complete stroke

Complete stroke (CVA) is diagnosed if neurological signs and symptoms last more than 24 hours. It is imperative to obtain medical care as soon as possible to improve outcome. Tissue Plasminogen Activator (tPA) should be started immediately if appropriate. It can only be given within 3 hours of symptoms starting to reduce the chance for long term disability. Approximately 5% of patients who have a transient ischemic attack will have a cerebrovascular accident within one month, and 30% of will have a cerebrovascular accident within one year.

Fainting

Syncope is fainting — a temporary loss of consciousness caused by a disruption in the blood flow to the brain. The insufficiency of blood results in a lack of oxygen in the brain. When the patient falls flat, blood flow to the brain is restored and the problem corrects itself. Put the patient in recovery position. Alert the doctor and phone EMS (911) if necessary.

Syncope may result from: Emotional stress; physical pain; standing in one position for too long; overheating; dehydration; exhaustion; rapid changes in blood pressure; heart disease; neurological disorders; lung disease; or an adverse reaction to medication. If syncope occurs with exercise or is associated with irregularities in heart rhythm, it can indicate a serious health problem. Sharp muscle contractions called myoclonic jerks may occur with syncope. This is not true seizure activity. Bradycardia and increased vagal tone are often seen in cases of syncope.

Wound type

Contusion

Contusion is a raised bruise (hematoma); treat contusions during the first 48 hours by applying cold packs for 15 minutes on and 15 minutes off, taking acetaminophen or ibuprofen, and elevating the area. Warm washcloths help after the second day.

Laceration

Laceration is a long break in the surface of the skin; the edges of a laceration may be linear (smooth) or stellate (irregular). A laceration is caused by a knife blow, glass, or a surgeon's scalpel and usually requires sutures.

Abrasion

Abrasion is a scrape or scratch of the outer layer of the skin; friction burns and rug burns are types of abrasions. Wash the wound and remove gravel with a forceps.

Avulsion

Avulsion is a flap of tissue that is torn away from the main body of tissue, which often requires sutures.

Puncture

Puncture is a small, deep perforation of the skin caused by teeth, needles, ice-picks, small caliber bullets, and other narrow, sharp objects. The doctor irrigates and probes the puncture.

Amputation

Amputation is when the body part is completely detached. Wrap the amputated part in a sterile dressing and place in a labeled plastic bag on ice. A surgeon may be able to reattach it.

Nutrition

Nutrients and blood production

Humans need the nutrients iron, folate, Vitamin B6 Vitamin B12, Vitamin C, Vitamin E, Vitamin K, riboflavin, copper, zinc, and protein to manufacture blood in the bone marrow. Even if these nutrients are adequate, the patient cannot produce sufficient blood without the hormone erythropoietin from the kidneys; patients with end-stage renal failure who are on dialysis become anemic.

Anemia is lack of blood or a deficiency in red blood cells. Signs and symptoms of anemia are fatigue, thirst, rapid pulse, pallor, dizziness, sweating, shortness of breath, abdominal or chest pain, leg cramps, and syncope.

Aplastic anemia results from suppressed bone marrow, due to leukemia, radiation or poisoning. Protein deficiency causes kwashiorkor anemia. Strict vegetarianism and chronic bleeding (e.g., heavy menstruation) deplete iron stores (ferritin), thereby causing iron deficiency anemia. Vitamin B12 deficiency causes pernicious anemia. Anemia occurs from increased red blood cell destruction from sickle-cell anemia, thalassemia, G6PD deficiency, autoimmune reaction, inherited disorders, hemolytic poison, or an enlarged spleen.

Fat-soluble vitamins

Vitamin A

Vitamin A (retinol) aids growth, development, immune function, and maintains night vision. Sources are butter, egg yolks, cod liver oil, yellow and green leafy vegetables, and prunes. Deficiency causes night blindness, poor visual acuity, skin disorders, and bronchopulmonary dysplasia in low birth weight newborns.

Vitamin D

Vitamin D(calciferol) aids calcium & phosphorus absorption for bone and teeth formation and necessary for normal growth and development. Sources are milk, cod liver oil, butter, and egg yolks. Sunlight activates Vitamin D. Deficiency causes rickets and osteomalacia (soft bones, bowed legs) and dental caries

Vitamin E

Vitamin E (tocopherols) is an antioxidant found in sunflower seeds, wheat germ, egg yolks, vegetable oils, almonds, olives, and papaya. Deficiency causes hemolytic anemia of premature newborns.

Vitamin K
Vitamin K (quinones) is a necessary for normal clotting of the blood and is found in green leafy vegetables, meat, dairy products, alfalfa, fishmeal, oats, wheat, and rye. Deficiency causes hemorrhagic disease of the newborn. Caution must be taken if anticoagulants are being used as this may affect how the clotting of the blood. There is no known toxicity.

The small intestine absorbs fat-soluble vitamins, so patients who have had bowel resections, cystic fibrosis or malabsorption may have deficiencies. Fat-soluble vitamins accumulate in fat and the liver, and can be toxic.

Water-soluble vitamins

Thiamin
Thiamin (B1) is found in whole grains, egg yolk, legumes, nuts, pork, and brewer's yeast. Deficiency causes beriberi, confusion, muscle weakness, poor growth.

Riboflavin
Riboflavin (B2) is in meat, whole grains, brewer's yeast, green vegetables, milk, and eggs. Deficiency causes growth retardation, cracked mouth, and light sensitivity.

Niacin
Niacin (B3) is found in meat, fish and poultry, whole grains, dairy products, brewer's yeast, and legumes.

Deficiency causes pellagra, dermatitis, and malabsorption.

Pantothenate
Pantothenate (B5) is found in cheese and dairy products, , eggs, peanuts, beef, fish, legumes, and soy. Deficiency causes dermatitis and depression.

Pyridoxine
Pyridoxine (B6) is in whole grains, nuts, legumes, eggs, meat, fish, bran, and yeast. Deficiency causes dermatitis, cracked mouth, insomnia, weakness, irritability, a strange gait, and seizures.

Cobalamin
Cobalamin (B12) is in liver, milk, and eggs. Deficiency causes pernicious anemia. Loss of balance and nerve damage.

Biotin
Biotin (B7) is in egg yolks, liver, brewer's yeast and royal jelly.

Folic acid
Deficiency is rare Folic acid (B9) is in green, leafy vegetables, organ meat, beef, and whole grains and cereals, and legumes. Deficiency causes anemia, neural tube defects.

Ascorbic acid
Ascorbic acid (C) is found in citrus fruits, strawberries, melon and vegetables such as broccoli, peppers, tomatoes, potatoes, and green leafy. Deficiency causes scurvy, pyorrhea, bleeding gums, tooth and bone defects, and poor wound healing.

Seven macrominerals

The seven macrominerals are:
- Calcium for muscle contraction, conduction of nerve impulses, bone and tooth maintenance, and blood clotting
- Phosphorous for energy transfer, pH balance, and bone and tooth maintenance
- Sodium for fluid balance, function of nerves and muscles
- Potassium for fluid balance in the blood, acid-base balance, muscle building, and protein synthesis
- Chloride for pH balance and needed for digestive juices
- Sulfur, an essential component of protein that helps energy metabolism
- Magnesium for energy metabolism, muscle function, enzymes, and protein synthesis

Important trace minerals include:
- Chromium for metabolism of fats and carbohydrate
- Cobalt for red blood cell maintenance; Copper for blood, nerves, bones, and immune function; Fluoride to strengthen bones and teeth
- Iodine for thyroid function and metabolism; Iron to make red blood cells and protein; Manganese for formation of connective and skeletal tissue, reproduction, growth and metabolism; Molybdenum helps breakdown sulfites, nitrogen metabolism, enzyme function
- Selenium to protect against free radicals
- Zinc for immune response and tissue growth, wound healing

Dietary restrictions

Patients with dietary restrictions for medical reasons have diabetes, food allergies, missing digestive organs, end-stage renal disease (ESRD), phenylketonuria (PKU), or are taking MAO inhibitors for depression. The patients who have dietary restrictions for religious reasons include: Arabs, Jews, Hindus, and Seventh Day Adventists.

TPN

Many end-stage patients report anorexia (lack of appetite) and changes in the taste of food from medications, disease, or treatments. Anorexia means decreased food consumption, problems meeting the patient's nutritional needs, and distress for the patient's family. Total parenteral nutrition (TPN) replaces all or some of the patient's food with liquid nutrients delivered through a surgically implanted catheter in the subclavian vein under the collarbone, or jugular vein of the neck, or umbilical vein in the abdomen, or PICC line in the arm.

TPN can be given over the course of the day or overnight depending upon the patient's condition. A TPN bag will range in size from 500 to 3000 mL and requires an infusion pump and IV pole to administer. TPN must be provided under sterile conditions to reduce the risk for infection. There are many complications that can be associated with TPN including clotting issues, infection, and liver disease. Close monitoring by the health-care team is essential. TPN can cause discord in the family and ethical issues for caregivers because it prolongs life artificially. TPN removes the patient's pleasure and sense of normalcy from eating.

Ordering meal modifications

When the doctor admits your patient to hospital, rehab, or hospice, check the chart for known allergies, religion, and other conditions that may affect eating. For example, patients with alcoholism and liver disease and nursing mothers may need extra calories and supplements, whereas patients with diabetes and PKU have dietary restrictions. Flag this information to alert the dietitian and nurse at the receiving facility by checking off the appropriate boxes on the meal card and admitting forms.

You can find the nearest Registered Dietitian (RD), evidence-based medicine, and billing information through the American Dietetic Association at http://www.eatright.org/. If your patient is newly diagnosed with a significant digestive disorder (e.g., diabetes, celiac, or cancer), you can download reliable dietary handouts for him/her in English, Spanish, or Chinese from The Nutrition Care Manual at http://www.nutritioncaremanual.org/, if your facility subscribes to it.

Dysphagia

Esophageal dysphagia is difficulty swallowing. It is distinct from odynophagia, which is painful swallowing. Dysphagia can result from:

- Strictures, tumors or foreign bodies
- Motility disorders, including achalasia
- Spasms of the esophagus

Patients present with difficulty swallowing, choking or coughing during eating, chronic weight loss and aspiration pneumonia. The doctor diagnoses the cause of dysphagia with endoscopy, barium swallow and monometric studies of the esophagus.

Patients with stroke, Parkinson's disease, multiple sclerosis, Lou Gehrig's disease, myasthenia gravis, muscular dystrophy, and various palsies are prone to dysphagia in their end stages. The treatment approach depends on the underlying cause of the dysphagia, and may include physiotherapy to retrain swallowing muscles, acid blocking medications, surgery to remove obstructions, or placement of a gastrostomy tube.

Practice Test

Test Questions

1. What does the term edema mean? (pg. 9)
   a. Rash
   b. Within
   c. Vomiting
   d. Swelling

2. What is the appropriate way to take a radial pulse? (pg. 92)
   a. Place your index finger and middle finger on the wrist, under the pinky finger.
   b. Place your index finger and middle finger on the wrist, under the thumb.
   c. Place your thumb on the side of the neck, next to the trachea.
   d. Place your index finger on the inner side of the upper arm, about halfway between the shoulder and the elbow.

3. A patient is anxious and begins hyperventilating. His hands and lips start to feel numb and tingly, and he feels lightheaded. What is the physiological cause of his symptoms? (pg. 14 - 15)
   a. Excess carbon dioxide in the blood
   b. Excess oxygen in the blood
   c. Lack of carbon dioxide in the blood
   d. Lack of oxygen in the blood

4. Which of the following is NOT one of the five stages of grief as described by the Kübler-Ross model? (pg. 21)
   a. Delusions
   b. Anger
   c. Denial
   d. Bargaining

5. Which of the following is tracked on a standard growth chart for patients ages 2 to 20?
   a. Age, weight, BMI
   b. Age, head circumference, height
   c. Age, height, and weight
   d. Age, head circumference, weight, height

6. A patient is upset and angry after an appointment. She is distraught and unable to pay attention when you tell her what dates are available for her follow-up appointment. This results in some confusion, and the patient accuses you of not listening. What form of defense mechanism is this patient likely demonstrating?
    a. Displacement
    b. Projection
    c. Reaction formation
    d. Denial

7. You are asked to give a three-year-old child a dose of acetaminophen (Tylenol). The child weighs 15 kg. The medication order says to give the child a dose of 15 mg/kg. The oral solution concentration is 160 mg/5 mL. What dose of the oral solution should you give the child?
    a. 9 mL
    b. 5 mL
    c. 2 mL
    d. 7 mL

8. You have finished all of your assigned tasks and are thinking of leaving a few minutes early for your lunch break when the doctor approaches you and tells you that there are patients waiting to be seen, but the exam rooms have not yet been cleaned after the last patients. You know that this is the responsibility of another medical assistant in the office, but she is on the phone dealing with an important personal problem. What should you do?
    a. Explain to the doctor that cleaning the patient exam rooms isn't your assignment today, and tell the doctor where to find the appropriate medical assistant.
    b. Reassure the doctor that you will take care of the problem, and then quickly clean the rooms yourself.
    c. Wait until the other medical assistant is off the phone, and then tell her that the rooms need to be cleaned quickly.
    d. Ask someone else in the office to clean the patient exam rooms.

9. How should you position yourself in an exam room with a patient who seems angry and potentially aggressive?
    a. Position yourself between the patient and the door.
    b. Position yourself with a desk between you and the patient.
    c. Position yourself seated next to the patient.
    d. Position yourself as far as possible away from the patient.

10. How should electrocardiogram (ECG) chest leads be placed?
   a. V1: second intercostal space, just right of the sternum. V2: second intercostal space, just left of the sternum. V4: fifth intercostal space, midclavicular line. V3: halfway between leads V2 and V4. V5: fifth intercostal space, anterior axillary line. V6: fifth intercostal space, midaxillary line.
   b. V1: fourth intercostal space, just right of the sternum. V2: fourth intercostal space, just left of the sternum. V4: fifth intercostal space, midclavicular line. V3: halfway between leads V2 and V4. V5: below rib cage, anterior axillary line. V6: below rib cage, midaxillary line.
   c. V1: fourth intercostal space, just right of the sternum. V2: fourth intercostal space, just left of the sternum. V4: fifth intercostal space, midclavicular line. V3: halfway between leads V2 and V4. V5: fifth intercostal space, anterior axillary line. V6: fifth intercostal space, midaxillary line.
   d. V1: fourth intercostal space, just right of the sternum. V2: fourth intercostal space, just left of the sternum. V4: fourth intercostal space, midclavicular line. V3: halfway between leads V2 and V4. V5: fourth intercostal space, anterior axillary line. V6: fourth intercostal space, midaxillary line.

11. You witness a patient suddenly collapse in the office. You run to the patient and realize she is unconscious, does not have a pulse, and is not breathing. While someone else calls 911, you and your coworkers begin cardiopulmonary resuscitation (CPR). At what point should you use an automated external defibrillator (AED)?
   a. After one round or two minutes of CPR have been performed
   b. As soon as emergency medical help arrives
   c. If the patient still has no pulse after five minutes of CPR
   d. As soon as possible

12. What is the definition of active listening? (pg. 26)
   a. Taking careful notes while listening to the patient in order to record important data
   b. Listening for certain key terms that will help you to quickly identify the main points that the patient is making
   c. Listening to the patient and then responding by using paraphrasing to demonstrate understanding
   d. Making use of the time during which the patient is talking to formulate your next question

13. Which of the following would be appropriate to leave in a phone message for a patient?
   a. "I am calling to let you know that your test results are positive."
   b. "I am calling for Mr. Smith from the office of Dr. Brown."
   c. "I am calling to let you know that your prescription for amoxicillin has been called into your pharmacy."
   d. "I am calling for Mr. Smith about his recent visit to Dr. Brown about his cough."

14. Which of the following is NOT a requirement to be a certified medical assistant (CMA)?
   a. Completion of an accredited medical assisting program
   b. Passing the CMA certification examination
   c. Recertification of CMA credentials every 60 months
   d. Work at least 10 hours per week to maintain certification

15. Which of the following would NOT be included in a living will?
   a. Whether a patient would like cardiopulmonary resuscitation (CPR) if cardiac arrest occurs
   b. If a patient would like to be kept alive with life-prolonging equipment
   c. If a patient does not want to have tube feeding
   d. How a person's assets should be distributed

16. Which of the following is considered to be one of the best overall ways to prevent the spread of infection?
   a. Always wearing gloves
   b. Thorough hand washing
   c. Wearing a respiratory mask
   d. Wearing a protective gown

17. A patient requests that you send her health records to a new physician that she is seeing. Which of the following measures should you take to follow medical privacy guidelines?
   a. Call the other physician's office to make sure they are actually seeing the patient.
   b. Ask the physician you are working with to sign a form giving permission for you to send the records to the new physician.
   c. Have the patient sign a form agreeing to the release of the medical records to the new physician.
   d. Counsel the patient that it would be safer to not have her records sent to the new physician.

18. You are working as a medical assistant for a large group of physicians. The office is located in an ethnically diverse area, and a significant portion of the patient population does not speak English. You are asked to take the vital signs and initial history of a patient who only speaks a language that you do not know. Which of the following is the best action to take?
   a. Use the patient's nine-year-old son, who does speak English, as a translator.
   b. Use hand gestures in order to communicate with the patient.
   c. Use a translator phone service in order to communicate with the patient.
   d. Use an online translator to write the patient a note explaining that they need to come back with someone who speaks English.

19. Which of the following is NOT a correct way to handle biohazardous waste?
    a. Dispose of sharps such as glass or needles in a sharps container.
    b. Place biohazardous materials in white plastic trash bags.
    c. Sanitize biohazard waste containers if they become soiled.
    d. Make sure that biohazard waste containers are all labeled with the international biohazard symbol.

20. What should you do if you become aware that a colleague is working while intoxicated?
    a. Approach the colleague and warn them not to do it again.
    b. Report the situation to your supervisor.
    c. Make sure the colleague enters an appropriate treatment program.
    d. Tell your other coworkers so you can work as a group to ensure that the colleague is able to perform his or her job sufficiently.

21. When food is traveling through the gastrointestinal system, what part of the small intestine does it enter immediately after leaving the stomach?
    a. Jejunum
    b. Duodenum
    c. Ileum
    d. Rectum

22. A six-month-old baby in the waiting room suddenly begins to choke on a small toy. The baby's mother yells for help. You run into the room to assist and see that the baby is still conscious, but she is unable to cough or make crying noises. What steps should you take to try to relieve the obstruction?
    a. Lay the infant on the ground and give quick, consecutive thrusts on the middle of the breastbone with two fingers. After every 30 compressions, try to visualize the object that is blocking the airway.
    b. Open the baby's mouth and sweep your finger into the back of her throat to try to dislodge the obstructing object.
    c. Lay the infant face-down along your arm, cradling her jaw in your fingers. Using the palm of your other hand, give the baby five quick, firm blows on the back between the shoulder blades. Then, turn the infant face-up and give five quick thrusts on the middle of the breastbone with two fingers.
    d. Hold the infant on your lap, facing away from you. Use your fist to forcefully press inward and upward just under the breastbone.

23. A patient comes into the clinic complaining of weight loss, anxiety, sweating, and diarrhea. She is diagnosed with hyperthyroidism. The thyroid gland is part of what body system?
    a. Nervous system
    b. Musculoskeletal system
    c. Digestive system
    d. Endocrine system

24. If you are asked to give the patient a referral to a cardiac specialist, what should you do?
    a. Give the patient the name and contact information of a cardiac specialist who will see him for his problem.
    b. Tell the patient to look up which cardiologists are on his insurance plan and to make an appointment with one of them as soon as possible.
    c. Send the patient's chart to a cardiologist to see if the doctor would be interested in seeing the patient.
    d. Have the patient go to the closest hospital immediately and ask to be seen by a cardiologist.

25. A patient has just been started on warfarin, and you are asked to give her further instructions on dietary guidelines that she needs to be aware of while on this medication. Which of the following is an important dietary guideline to instruct the patient about?
    a. Maintain a consistent diet.
    b. Avoid eating green, leafy vegetables.
    c. Avoid drinking grapefruit juice.
    d. Eat double the recommended daily dose of fiber.

26. Which of the following is obesity LEAST likely to play a role in?
    a. Osteoporosis
    b. Gallstones
    c. Osteoarthritis
    d. Type II diabetes

27. Which of the following locations will yield the most accurate results when taking an infant's temperature?
    a. Mouth
    b. Armpit
    c. Rectum
    d. Ear

28. What does third-party medical billing refer to? (pg. 63)
    a. When a physician sends a bill to an insurance company
    b. When an insurance company contracts with another company to process payments
    c. When a patient has two separate forms of health insurance
    d. When a patient's insurance company handles a claim

29. If a patient is lying on their back, they are in a _____ position.
    a. Prone
    b. Prostrate
    c. Dorsal
    d. Supine

30. You are assisting a physician as he sutures a patient wound, and you inadvertently receive a needle stick. The needle had already been used on the patient, and it is therefore potentially contaminated. What action should be taken immediately?
    a. Irrigate the puncture wound.
    b. Get a tetanus shot.
    c. Call risk management.
    d. Begin HIV prophylaxis.

31. Which of the following is a federal guideline for protecting health information?
    a. HIPAA   (pg. 27)
    b. FMLA
    c. CSA
    d. HHS

32. What is the proper way to position a blood pressure cuff?
    a. Wrap the cuff loosely around the upper part of the forearm, about an inch below the elbow.
    b. Wrap the cuff snugly around the upper arm, as close to the shoulder as possible.
    c. Wrap the cuff around the elbow, just tight enough to keep it in place.
    d. Wrap the cuff snugly around the upper arm, about half an inch above the elbow.

33. Which of the following is an important and possibly life-threatening side effect of clopidogrel (Plavix)?
    a. Seizures
    b. Heart attack
    c. Bleeding
    d. Hypertension

34. Which of the following describes the correct sizing of crutches for a patient?
　　a. The top of the crutches should be six inches below the armpits when the patient is standing up straight, and the handgrips should be at the level of the hips.
　　b. The top of the crutches should be two inches below the armpits when the patient is standing up straight, and the handgrips should be at the level of the waist.
　　c. The top of the crutches should be one inch below the armpits when the patient is standing up straight, and the handgrips should be even with the top of the hips.
　　d. The top of the crutches should be four inches below the armpits when the patient is standing up straight. The handgrips can be positioned wherever the patient would like them.

35. What information should be recorded on all patient visit notes?
　　a. Time and date
　　b. Patient signature
　　c. Patient Social Security number
　　d. Physician's provider number

36. What does the prefix dys- mean?
　　a. Discharge
　　b. Around
　　c. Difficult
　　d. After

37. You are asked to collect a throat swab from a patient suspected of having strep throat. How should you carry out this procedure?
　　a. Have the patient open his mouth just enough to fit the swab in, then move the swab back and forth until you hit the back of the throat.
　　b. Depress the tongue, visualize the back of the throat, then swab the back of the throat and tonsils from side to side.
　　c. Clearly visualize the back of the throat, and only take a throat swab if there are white patches visible on the tonsils.
　　d. Depress the tongue, have the patient open his mouth wide, and then swab the throat, cheeks, and tongue.

38. Which of the following is NOT required to be on the label of a medical specimen?
　　a. Date of collection
　　b. Time of collection
　　c. The patient's full name
　　d. Full name and signature of the person collecting the specimen

39. Patients should not get the flu vaccine if they are allergic to what substance?
   a. Gluten
   b. Lactose
   c. Eggs
   d. Corn

40. If a patient is sitting with his arms crossed and the sides of his mouth slightly turned down while you are giving him instructions about a prescription, what would be an appropriate question to ask him?
   a. What is the problem?
   b. You don't like what I am saying?
   c. Do you want to do this appointment another time?
   d. Is there something that is bothering you?

41. What instructions should be given to a female patient when a clean-catch urine sample is needed?
   a. Use a sterile wipe to clean between the labial folds, wiping from back to front.
   b. Include the initial stream of urine in the sample.
   c. Do not allow the labial folds to become spread open.
   d. Urinate a small amount into the toilet bowl, then collect the sample using the urine cup.

42. Which of the following would be considered an open-ended question?
   a. What brings you to the office today?
   b. Are you feeling better?
   c. Is your leg pain still bothering you?
   d. Have you been experiencing nausea?

43. You are asked to take an elderly patient to get an x-ray of her chest. What should your role be in ensuring the patient's safety during the test?
   a. Make sure the patient is secured on the imaging table to reduce the risk of a fall.
   b. Hold the patient's arm during the x-ray to make sure she remains still.
   c. Check the settings on the x-ray equipment to make sure the radiation dose is correct.
   d. Make sure that the patient receives a dose of medicine for anxiety before the test.

44. What drug class does simvastatin (Zocor) belong to?
   a. Pain-relieving medications
   b. Cholesterol-lowering medications
   c. Hormone-replacement medications
   d. Antihypertensive medication

45. Which of the following is an appropriate site for an intramuscular injection?
   a. Triceps muscle
   b. Dorsogluteal muscle
   c. Quadriceps femoris muscle
   d. Soleus muscle

46. Which of the following classes of controlled substances has no currently accepted medical use in the United States?
   a. Schedule I controlled substances
   b. Schedule II controlled substances
   c. Schedule IV controlled substances
   d. Schedule V controlled substances

47. Which of the following actions does NOT help prevent the contamination of blood samples?
   a. Wiping the shaft of the needle used to draw the blood sample with an alcohol swab
   b. Disinfecting the patient's skin in the area the blood is to be drawn
   c. Washing your hands before drawing the blood sample
   d. Wearing gloves

48. Which of the following are appropriate steps when giving a nebulizer treatment to a patient? (pg. 71)
   a. Check the patient's armband and/or ask the patient to verify his or her identification, check the physician's order to ensure that the correct type and dose of medication are being used, have the patient hold the face mask four to six inches away from his or her mouth, and instruct the patient to take deep breaths of the medicated vapor until the medication has been fully dispensed.
   b. Check the patient's armband and/or ask the patient to verify his or her identification, check the physician's order to ensure that the correct type and dose of medication are being used, place the face mask securely over the patient's mouth and nose, and instruct the patient to take very shallow breaths of the medicated vapor until the medication has been fully dispensed.
   c. Check the patient's armband and/or ask the patient to verify his or her identification, check the physician's order to ensure that the correct type and dose of medication are being used, place the face mask securely over the patient's mouth and nose, and instruct the patient to take deep breaths of the medicated vapor until the medication has been fully dispensed.
   d. Check the patient's armband and/or ask the patient to verify his or her identification, check the physician's order for the appropriate type and dose of medication, place double the amount of the ordered medication in the nebulizer cup because only about half of it will end up being inhaled by the patient, place the face mask securely over the patient's mouth and nose, and instruct the patient to take deep breaths of the medicated vapor until the medication has been fully dispensed.

49. A patient runs into the office while you are in the reception area alone. He is bleeding severely from a wound to the leg. After calling for help, what should you do immediately to help the patient?

a. Apply direct and continuous pressure to the wound with a clean cloth or bandage.

b. Apply a tourniquet three to four inches above the wound, and pull it tight until the bleeding stops.

c. Wash the wound well with sterile water, and then apply a secure bandage.

d. Squeeze the main artery in the groin area to prevent more blood from being delivered to the lower leg.

50. What are standard precautions?

a. Guidelines about protecting yourself from a potentially aggressive patient

b. Guidelines about how to set up an office for patient and employee safely

c. Guidelines about how to prevent patients from suing

d. Guidelines about protecting yourself from potential infection

Answers and Explanations

1. D: The term edema means swelling. The swelling is caused by an accumulation of fluid within the tissues of the body. Exanthema refers to a rash. The prefix endo- means within. The suffix -emesis refers to vomiting.

2. B: The radial pulse is palpated at the wrist, under the thumb. When taking a pulse, you should use the pads of your index finger and middle finger. Your thumb has a pulse beat of its own, which may interfere with feeling the patient's pulse. The carotid pulse is palpated on the side of the neck, next to the trachea. The brachial pulse is palpated on the inner side of the upper arm, about halfway between the shoulder and elbow. The ulnar artery pulse is located at the wrist, under the pinky, but it is not as commonly used as the radial pulse.

3. C: Hyperventilation refers to a patient breathing more quickly than normal. This rapid rate of ventilation results in carbon dioxide being exhaled at a higher rate than normal. This can result in metabolic alkalosis, meaning that the pH of the blood is abnormally elevated. The symptoms that may accompany hyperventilation are related to the metabolic alkalosis that develops. The patient should be reassured in a calm manner to reduce anxiety. Have the patient sit down and instruct him to take slow, deep breaths.

4. A: The five stages of grief, as listed in the popular Kübler-Ross model, include denial, anger, bargaining, depression, and acceptance. These stages of grief may be experienced by a person facing death or by his or her survivors. They may be experienced in any order. Not everyone experiences all five stages, and some people experience other emotions not listed here. Delusions are beliefs that are held very strongly despite the fact that they are clearly false. They reflect an abnormal thought process and may be present in certain mental disorders.

5. C: Growth charts are used to track a child's growth over time. On a standard growth chart, the patient's height and weight are measured and charted according to the patient's age. Body mass index (BMI) charts may also be used, with BMI being calculated from the measured height and weight. Under usual circumstances, head circumference is not tracked in toddlers and older children. The important part of the chart is the overall pattern of growth and rate of change.

6. B: Projection is when a patient attributes their own undesired thoughts, feelings, or actions to another person. For instance, this upset patient is not listening or paying attention when you try to help her set up an appointment. She becomes more upset and then accuses you of not listening, when she is actually the one who is not listening. Displacement is when thoughts or feelings about one person are taken out on another person or object. Reaction formation is when a person converts

unwanted feelings or thoughts into their opposites. Denial is when a person will not accept reality.

7. D: The child weighs 15 kg and needs to receive 15 mg of acetaminophen for every kg of body weight. The total dose should equal 225 mg (15 kg x 15 mg/kg = 225 mg). Because you know there are 160 mg/5 mL, you can calculate that there are 32 mg in every mL. In order to find out the dose in mL, divide 225 mg by 32 mg/mL, which equals 7 mL.

8. B: Teamwork is an important part of any medical career. Being willing to work as a team will help keep things running smoothly when unexpected issues arise. As part of a medical team, you will be expected to work with others to take care of patients in a safe and competent manner. In a professional work environment, you should be willing to help your coworkers when the need arises.

9. A: If you are faced with a potentially aggressive patient, it is recommended that you make sure that you are positioned between the patient and the door so you can rapidly leave the room, if necessary.

10. C: The correct placement is as described in answer C. It is important to place the leads correctly and precisely so that the electrocardiogram (ECG) can be correctly interpreted. V1 and V2 give information about the right side of the heart. V3 and V4 give information about the interventricular septum. V5 and V6 give information about the left side of the heart.

11. D: Because you witnessed the collapse of the patient, the automated external defibrillator (AED) should be used as soon as possible. The AED will evaluate the patient's heart rhythm while cardiopulmonary resuscitation (CPR) is being performed, so CPR can be continued while the AED pads are being applied if there is more than one responder present. The AED will give step-by-step instructions and indicate whether the patient needs to be shocked or whether CPR alone should be continued. If a patient is found unconscious and the collapse was not witnessed, two minutes or one round of CPR should be performed before using the AED.

12. C: Active listening has been found to be a useful and empathetic way to communicate with patients. It involves listening carefully to what the patient is telling you and then restating what the patient has said back to him or her. This not only ensures that you correctly understand what the patient is saying, but it also demonstrates to the patient that they are being heard.

13. B: When leaving a phone message for a patient, you can identify who the message is for and identify yourself and the office. You can then ask the patient to return the call. You should not leave any medical information, including test results or prescription drug names, in a phone message.

14. D: In order to be a certified medical assistant (CMA), the applicant must complete an accredited medical assisting program, pass the CMA certification examination, and recertify his or her credentials every 60 months. In addition, the applicant must maintain current, provider-level CPR certification. The number of hours worked per week is not a specified requirement to be a CMA.

15. D: A living will is a written document that specifies what a patient would like to be done if he becomes unable to make healthcare decisions for himself. In a living will, the patient can express his wishes about what life-prolonging treatments he wants or does not want under various circumstances. It is a document focused on healthcare decisions, not on the patient's material assets.

16. B: Healthcare workers should thoroughly wash their hands before and after each patient contact. The Centers for Disease Control and Prevention (CDC) considers hand washing as one of the best ways to prevent the spread of infection. Hands should be washed with warm water and soap and should be vigorously rubbed together for at least 20 seconds. You should be sure to clean the back of your hands, under your nails, between your fingers, and your wrists. Hand sanitizers are another option, but they do not work as well as hand washing.

17. C: Patient records cannot be sent to other providers without the patient's consent. In order to be protected legally, you should have the patient sign an authorization form for the release of her medical records to the other physician. Ideally, this form would include a description of the information that will be released, the name and contact information of the recipient, a statement that the patient understands what will be disclosed, and the signature of the patient. It is not necessary for you to call the new physician or to have the physician you are working for sign a permission form. It can be very helpful and important for all of a patient's physicians to have access to the patient's previous medical records, so counseling the patient to not send the records would be inappropriate.

18. C: Ideally, you would use a translator phone service in order to communicate with the patient. Using the translator phone, you can explain to the patient what you need to do to take his or her vital signs and then ask the necessary questions for the initial patient history. In a large practice that has a diverse patient population or in a hospital setting, this type of service is often available. If the patient's young child is asked to translate, a number of problems may arise. There would be issues with patient privacy, potential problems with translation accuracy, and possible embarrassment for the parent and child. Hand gestures may be necessary, but would not be as useful as a translator phone. Asking the patient to come back with a translator should be avoided if possible.

19. B: Biohazard bags are generally red and should be labeled with the word "Biohazard" along with the international biohazard symbol. All sharps should be disposed of in appropriate sharps containers that are rigid and puncture resistant. If

a biohazard container becomes soiled, guidelines should be followed to sanitize the container.

20. B: Ethically and legally, it is your duty to protect your patients. If a colleague is coming to work while intoxicated, this could place patients at risk. You should report the situation to your supervisor so appropriate action can be taken. An intoxicated employee should not be working with patients.

21. B: The small intestine is divided into three major parts. The duodenum is the first section, just distal to the stomach; the jejunum is the middle section; and the ileum is the third section that connects to the large intestine.

22. C: Answer C describes the correct way to provide choking first aid to a conscious child under the age of one. You continue to repeat the five back blows and five chest thrusts until the object is dislodged or until the baby becomes unconscious. Answer A describes infant CPR, which is what should be done if the choking baby becomes unconscious. You should not perform blind finger sweeps, as described in B because this may push the object further into the throat. If you can visualize the object, you can try to reach in and pull it out. Answer D describes how you would do the Heimlich maneuver in an older child or adult.

23. D: The endocrine system consists of a group of glands that secretes hormones into the blood. These hormones play important roles in regulating various functions of the body. With hyperthyroidism, there is excess thyroid hormone being secreted by the thyroid gland, and this can cause a number of symptoms, including weight loss, anxiety, sweating, and diarrhea.

24. A: If asked to give a patient a referral, you should give the patient the name and contact information of the type of doctor they need to see. Ideally, you will check and make sure that the referral physician takes the patient's insurance and is taking new patients, or you can tell the patient to check before his visit. Sometimes you may even make an appointment for the patient with the referral doctor. Having the patient find a doctor to see on his own is not giving him a referral. Sending the patient's chart to the specialist to see if he or she would be interested in taking the case would breach the patient's privacy, and is not how referrals are made.

25. A: The most important dietary guideline to tell patients about when starting warfarin is that it is important to be consistent with their diets. Foods high in vitamin K, such as green leafy vegetables, can alter the effects of warfarin therapy, but as long as the patient is consistent in the intake of these foods, the medication can be adjusted accordingly.

26. A: Obesity is associated with numerous health problems. These include gallstones, osteoarthritis, type II diabetes, heart disease, hypertension, and various types of cancer. It was previously thought that obese patients were LESS likely to

have osteoporosis than nonobese patients, but new research is questioning this theory. Obesity has been directly linked to the other listed health problems, but research is still ongoing about the association between obesity and osteoporosis.

27. C: A rectal temperature reading is considered the most accurate for infants. Other methods can be used to take an infant's temperature, but it is important to get the most accurate reading as possible in infants because their health is generally more delicate than that of older children. The closer the thermometer is to the inside of the body, the warmer and more accurate the temperature will be.

28. B: Third-party medical billing companies are companies that are used by insurance companies to process claims or payments. The physician may submit a claim to an insurance company, and the insurance company then passes the claim on to another company that specializes in processing that type of claims.

29. D: The definition of supine is lying on the back with the face upward or having the palm of the hand facing upward. Prone is the position of lying on the stomach or having the palm of the hand facing downward. Dorsal refers to the back of the body. Prostrate is defined as being stretched out, face-down.

30. A: If you receive a needle stick, you should immediately irrigate the wound with a large amount of sterile saline or another clean fluid. A tetanus shot may be necessary depending on your vaccination status, but it can be given after you irrigate the wound. After irrigating the wound, your supervisor should be informed and you should be evaluated to determine what other tests and vaccinations are necessary. It is possible that you may need prophylaxis for human immunodeficiency virus (HIV), but this can also be done after you have washed the wound.

31. A: The Health Insurance Portability and Accountability Act (HIPAA) is a federal act that addresses the privacy of personal health information. It provides details about how personal health information must be protected.

32. D: A blood pressure cuff should ideally be placed on the upper arm, about half an inch above the elbow. The blood pressure cuff should be wrapped snugly around the arm in order to achieve proper compression of the brachial artery. You should be able to fit one finger underneath the cuff. If the cuff is too tight or too loose, the blood pressure reading may be inaccurate. Many cuffs have a brachial artery marker, which indicates how the cuff should be positioned on the arm (with the brachial artery marker just above the inner crease of the elbow).

33. C: Severe bleeding is a serious potential side effect of Plavix. Plavix is a blood thinner that is used therapeutically to prevent blood clots in high-risk patients. All patients on this medication and all healthcare providers should be aware that bleeding is one of the major risk factors associated with Plavix.

34. C: The top of the crutches should be 1 to 1.5 inches below the armpits when the patient is standing up straight. The handgrips should be even with the top of the patient's hips. It is important to size crutches correctly for a patient to avoid putting stress on other parts of the body. Improper sizing may result in discomfort and potential injury.

35. A: The correct time and date should be recorded on all patient documents. In addition, often the patient's name, birth date, and medical record number are included on documents. There are several types of documents that do require the patient's signature, Social Security number, and other personal information, but this information is not required on *all* patient visit documentation. The physician's provider number is used for health insurance purposes, and it is not required to be written on all patient visit notes.

36. C: The prefix dys- means abnormal or difficult. Examples include dysphagia, which means difficulty swallowing, and dysplasia, which means the abnormal growth of tissues or cells. The suffix -rrhea means discharge. The prefix peri- means around. The prefix post- means after.

37. B: Have the patient open his mouth wide and tilt back his head. Use a tongue depressor to depress the patient's tongue so you can see the back of the throat. Swab the back of the throat and over the tonsils from side to side. Make sure you swab any visible white patches or inflamed areas in the throat and tonsils. Avoid swabbing the tongue and cheeks because you want to focus on the bacteria collected from the throat and tonsillar area. Even if white patches are not seen on the tonsils, the patient still may have a bacterial infection and a throat swab should be taken.

38. D: When labeling medical specimens (e.g., blood, urine, or sputum) it is important to include the date and time of collection, the type of specimen, and the patient's full name and date of birth or medical record number. Although the full name and signature of the person collecting the specimen are not required, the collector should include his or her initials on the label.

39. C: The flu vaccine is grown in eggs. If a patient is allergic to eggs, he or she may have an allergic reaction to the flu vaccine. Other contraindications for the flu vaccine are a previous history of allergic reaction to the vaccine, a history of Guillain–Barré syndrome, or the patient currently has a fever.

40. D: Many times patients may communicate in nonverbal ways, such as using body language. It is important to pay attention to these cues because this may help you to better understand and respond to your patient. In this case, a patient who is frowning with his arms folded may indicate that he disapproves of something, does not accept what you are saying, or has another issue. When a patient displays nonverbal cues, you can use these to considerately question the patient about his

feelings. Asking, "What is the problem?" would be an abrupt and possibly rude way to approach the patient. Asking, "You don't like what I am saying?" or "Do you want to do this appointment another time?" may be overinterpreting the patient's feelings.

41. D: When a clean-catch urine sample is needed from a female patient, she should be instructed to sit on the toilet, spread open the labial folds with two fingers, use a sterile wipe to clean the inner folds of the labia (wiping from front to back), and use a second wipe to clean the area over the urethra. The patient should then urinate a small amount into the toilet bowl, temporarily stop the flow of urine, and then collect a urine sample using the urine cup.

42. A: Open-ended questions are those that encourage the patient to give full answers in their own words. Close-ended questions often result in one-word answers, and therefore they may not result in as much information being provided. It is important to use open-ended questions when performing medical interviews so the patient can give meaningful and detailed answers.

43. A: When accompanying a patient to other parts of the clinic or hospital for testing, it is important to ensure that the patient remains safe and comfortable. It is your responsibility to safely transport your patient and make sure that she is securely on the imaging table to prevent falls. In general, you will be in another room when the x-ray is taken to reduce your own exposure to the radiation. You should not hold onto the patient during the x-ray. It is the radiology technician's responsibility to ensure that the equipment settings are correct. In most cases, patients do not need anxiety medication before an x-ray is performed.

44. B: Simvastatin (Zocor) is a statin. Statins are 3-hydroxy-3-methyl coenzyme A (HMG-CoA) reductase inhibitors, which work to lower cholesterol.

45. B: The four sites most appropriate for intramuscular injections are the deltoid muscle, the vastus lateralis muscle, the ventrogluteal muscle, and the dorsogluteal muscle. The deltoid muscle is located in the upper arm. The vastus lateralis muscle is located in the thigh. The ventrogluteal muscle is located in the hip. The dorsogluteal muscle is the large muscle in the buttock. When selecting which site to use, you should consider the age of the patient, the medication that is being injected, and the general condition of the patient.

46. A: Schedule I controlled substances are drugs that have a very high potential for abuse and have no currently accepted medical use in the United States. Schedule II drugs also have a very high potential for abuse, but they have accepted medical uses. Schedule IV and V controlled substances have a lower potential for abuse compared to Schedule I through III substances.

47. A: The needles used for blood collection come in sterile packaging. After uncapping the needle, it is best to avoid touching its shaft (the part of the needle that will puncture the patient's skin). Wiping the needle with an alcohol swab is unnecessary because the needle is already sterile. Disinfecting the patient's skin, washing your hands, and wearing gloves will all help prevent contamination of blood samples.

48. C: It is important to always verify a patient's identification before giving any treatments. It is also essential to check that the correct type and dose of medication are being given, exactly as ordered by the physician. During a nebulizer treatment, the patient should have the face mask placed securely over his or her mouth and nose in order to ensure that the majority of the medication is inhaled. If the face mask is held several inches away, the medication may disperse into the air rather than being inhaled by the patient. The patient should be instructed to take deep breaths so the nebulized medication is carried into the lungs.

49. A: When a patient presents with severe bleeding from a wound, continuous pressure should be applied directly to the wound for at least 20 minutes. If the blood seeps through the bandage, more material should be added on top without taking off the first bandage. If applying direct pressure to the wound does not stop the bleeding, the main artery supplying the area can be occluded (at the "pressure point") by squeezing the artery against the bone. If a patient is bleeding severely, you should not take time to clean the wound, but first focus on stopping the bleeding. Applying a tourniquet should not be the immediate reaction to severe bleeding because this can have significant adverse effects.

50. D: Standard precautions are a set of medical practice guidelines that are meant to protect healthcare workers from infection. Healthcare workers are instructed to use standard precautions to prevent contact with blood and all other potentially infectious substances. In any situation where they may be exposed to bodily fluids (e.g., blood, cerebral spinal fluid, vaginal secretions), employees should wear personal protective equipment (e.g., gloves, masks, gowns, and eye protection) and wash their hands. These guidelines apply to the care of all patients, regardless of status.

Secret Key #1 – Time is Your Greatest Enemy

To succeed on the GACE, you must use your time wisely. Many students do not finish at least one section. The time constraints are brutal. To succeed, you must ration your time properly.

Pace Yourself

Wear a watch. At the beginning of the test, check the time (or start a chronometer on your watch to count the minutes), and check the time after every few questions to make sure you are "on schedule."

If you are forced to speed up, do it efficiently. Usually one or more answer choices can be eliminated without too much difficulty. Above all, don't panic. Don't speed up and just begin guessing at random choices. By pacing yourself, and continually monitoring your progress against your watch, you will always know exactly how far ahead or behind you are with your available time. If you find that you are one minute behind on the test, don't skip one question without spending any time on it, just to catch back up. Take 15 fewer seconds on the next four questions, and after four questions you'll have caught back up. Once you catch back up, you can continue working each problem at your normal pace.

Furthermore, don't dwell on the problems that you were rushed on. If a problem was taking up too much time and you made a hurried guess, it must be difficult. The difficult questions are the ones you are most likely to miss anyway, so it isn't a big loss. It is better to end with more time than you need than to run out of time.

Lastly, sometimes it is beneficial to slow down if you are constantly getting ahead of time. You are always more likely to catch a careless mistake by working more slowly than quickly, and among very high-scoring test takers (those who are likely to have lots of time left over), careless errors affect the score more than mastery of material.

Secret Key #2 - Guessing is not Guesswork

You probably know that guessing is a good idea - unlike other standardized tests, there is no penalty for getting a wrong answer. Even if you have no idea about a question, you still have a 20-25% chance of getting it right.

Most test takers do not understand the impact that proper guessing can have on their score. Unless you score extremely high, guessing will significantly contribute to your final score.

Monkeys Take the Test

What most test takers don't realize is that to insure that 20-25% chance, you have to guess randomly. If you put 20 monkeys in a room to take this test, assuming they answered once per question and behaved themselves, on average they would get 20-25% of the questions correct. Put 20 test takers in the room, and the average will be much lower among guessed questions. Why?

1. The test writers intentionally writes deceptive answer choices that "look" right. A test taker has no idea about a question, so picks the "best looking" answer, which is often wrong. The monkey has no idea what looks good and what doesn't, so will consistently be lucky about 20-25% of the time.
2. Test takers will eliminate answer choices from the guessing pool based on a hunch or intuition. Simple but correct answers often get excluded, leaving a 0% chance of being correct. The monkey has no clue, and often gets lucky with the best choice.

This is why the process of elimination endorsed by most test courses is flawed and detrimental to your performance- test takers don't guess, they make an ignorant stab in the dark that is usually worse than random.

$5 Challenge

Let me introduce one of the most valuable ideas of this course- the $5 challenge:

You only mark your "best guess" if you are willing to bet $5 on it.
You only eliminate choices from guessing if you are willing to bet $5 on it.

Why $5? Five dollars is an amount of money that is small yet not insignificant, and can really add up fast (20 questions could cost you $100). Likewise, each answer choice on one question of the test will have a small impact on your overall score, but it can really add up to a lot of points in the end.

The process of elimination IS valuable. The following shows your chance of guessing it right:

If you eliminate wrong answer choices until only this many remain:	Chance of getting it correct:
1	100%
2	50%
3	33%

However, if you accidentally eliminate the right answer or go on a hunch for an incorrect answer, your chances drop dramatically: to 0%. By guessing among all the answer choices, you are GUARANTEED to have a shot at the right answer.

That's why the $5 test is so valuable- if you give up the advantage and safety of a pure guess, it had better be worth the risk.

What we still haven't covered is how to be sure that whatever guess you make is truly random. Here's the easiest way:
Always pick the first answer choice among those remaining.

Such a technique means that you have decided, before you see a single test question, exactly how you are going to guess- and since the order of choices tells you nothing about which one is correct, this guessing technique is perfectly random.

This section is not meant to scare you away from making educated guesses or eliminating choices- you just need to define when a choice is worth eliminating. The $5 test, along with a pre-defined random guessing strategy, is the best way to make sure you reap all of the benefits of guessing.

Secret Key #3 - Practice Smarter, Not Harder

Many test takers delay the test preparation process because they dread the awful amounts of practice time they think necessary to succeed on the test. We have refined an effective method that will take you only a fraction of the time.

There are a number of "obstacles" in your way to succeed. Among these are answering questions, finishing in time, and mastering test-taking strategies. All must be executed on the day of the test at peak performance, or your score will suffer. The test is a mental marathon that has a large impact on your future.

Just like a marathon runner, it is important to work your way up to the full challenge. So first you just worry about questions, and then time, and finally strategy:

Success Strategy

1. Find a good source for practice tests.
2. If you are willing to make a larger time investment, consider using more than one study guide- often the different approaches of multiple authors will help you "get" difficult concepts.
3. Take a practice test with no time constraints, with all study helps "open book." Take your time with questions and focus on applying strategies.

4. Take a practice test with time constraints, with all guides "open book."
5. Take a final practice test with no open material and time limits

If you have time to take more practice tests, just repeat step 5. By gradually exposing yourself to the full rigors of the test environment, you will condition your mind to the stress of test day and maximize your success.

Secret Key #4 - Prepare, Don't Procrastinate

Let me state an obvious fact: if you take the test three times, you will get three different scores. This is due to the way you feel on test day, the level of preparedness you have, and, despite the test writers' claims to the contrary, some tests WILL be easier for you than others.

Since your future depends so much on your score, you should maximize your chances of success. In order to maximize the likelihood of success, you've got to prepare in advance. This means taking practice tests and spending time learning the information and test taking strategies you will need to succeed.

Never take the test as a "practice" test, expecting that you can just take it again if you need to. Feel free to take sample tests on your own, but when you go to take the official test, be prepared, be focused, and do your best the first time!

Secret Key #5 - Test Yourself

Everyone knows that time is money. There is no need to spend too much of your time or too little of your time preparing for the test. You should only spend as much of your precious time preparing as is necessary for you to get the score you need.

Once you have taken a practice test under real conditions of time constraints, then you will know if you are ready for the test or not.

If you have scored extremely high the first time that you take the practice test, then there is not much point in spending countless hours studying. You are already there.

Benchmark your abilities by retaking practice tests and seeing how much you have improved. Once you score high enough to guarantee success, then you are ready. If you have scored well below where you need, then knuckle down and begin studying in earnest. Check your improvement regularly through the use of practice tests under real conditions. Above all, don't worry, panic, or give up. The key is perseverance!

Then, when you go to take the test, remain confident and remember how well you did on the practice tests. If you can score high enough on a practice test, then you can do the same on the real thing.

General Strategies

The most important thing you can do is to ignore your fears and jump into the test immediately- do not be overwhelmed by any strange-sounding terms. You have to jump into the test like jumping into a pool- all at once is the easiest way.

Make Predictions

As you read and understand the question, try to guess what the answer will be. Remember that several of the answer choices are wrong, and once you begin reading them, your mind will immediately become cluttered with answer choices designed to throw you off. Your mind is typically the most focused immediately after you have read the question and digested its contents. If you can, try to predict what the correct answer will be. You may be surprised at what you can predict.

Quickly scan the choices and see if your prediction is in the listed answer choices. If it is, then you can be quite confident that you have the right answer. It still won't hurt to check the other answer choices, but most of the time, you've got it!

Answer the Question

It may seem obvious to only pick answer choices that answer the question, but the test writers can create some excellent answer choices that are wrong. Don't pick an answer just because it sounds right, or you believe it to be true. It MUST answer the question. Once you've made your selection, always go back and check it against the question and make sure that you didn't misread the question, and the answer choice does answer the question posed.

Benchmark

After you read the first answer choice, decide if you think it sounds correct or not. If it doesn't, move on to the next answer choice. If it does, mentally mark that answer choice. This doesn't mean that you've definitely selected it as your answer choice, it just means that it's the best you've seen thus far. Go ahead and read the next choice. If the next choice is worse than the one you've already selected, keep going to the next answer choice. If the next choice is better than the choice you've already selected, mentally mark the new answer choice as your best guess.

The first answer choice that you select becomes your standard. Every other answer choice must be benchmarked against that standard. That choice is correct until proven otherwise by another answer choice beating it out. Once you've decided that no other answer choice seems as good, do one final check to ensure that your answer choice answers the question posed.

Valid Information

Don't discount any of the information provided in the question. Every piece of information may be necessary to determine the correct answer. None of the information in the question is there to throw you off (while the answer choices will certainly have information to throw you off). If two seemingly unrelated topics are discussed, don't ignore either. You can be confident there is a relationship, or it wouldn't be included in the question, and you are probably going to have to determine what is that relationship to find the answer.

Avoid "Fact Traps"

Don't get distracted by a choice that is factually true. Your search is for the answer that answers the question. Stay focused and don't fall for an answer that is true but incorrect. Always go back to the question and make sure you're choosing an answer that actually answers the question and is not just a true statement. An answer can be factually correct, but it MUST answer the question asked. Additionally, two answers can both be seemingly correct, so be sure to read all of the answer choices, and make sure that you get the one that BEST answers the question.

Milk the Question

Some of the questions may throw you completely off. They might deal with a subject you have not been exposed to, or one that you haven't reviewed in years. While your lack of knowledge about the subject will be a hindrance, the question itself can give you many clues that will help you find the correct answer. Read the question carefully and look for clues. Watch particularly for adjectives and nouns describing difficult terms or words that you don't recognize. Regardless of if you completely understand a word or not, replacing it with a synonym either provided or one you more familiar with may help you to understand what the questions are asking. Rather than wracking your mind about specific detailed information concerning a difficult term or word, try to use mental substitutes that are easier to understand.

The Trap of Familiarity

Don't just choose a word because you recognize it. On difficult questions, you may not recognize a number of words in the answer choices. The test writers don't put "make-believe" words on the test; so don't think that just because you only recognize all the words in one answer choice means that answer choice must be correct. If you only recognize words in one answer choice, then focus on that one. Is it correct? Try your best to determine if it is correct. If it is, that is great, but if it doesn't, eliminate it. Each word and answer choice you eliminate increases your chances of getting the question correct, even if you then have to guess among the unfamiliar choices.

Eliminate Answers

Eliminate choices as soon as you realize they are wrong. But be careful! Make sure you consider all of the possible answer choices. Just because one appears right, doesn't mean that the next one won't be even better! The test writers will usually put more than one good answer choice for every question, so read all of them. Don't worry if you are stuck between two that seem right. By getting down to just two remaining possible choices, your odds are now 50/50. Rather than wasting too much time, play the odds. You are guessing, but guessing wisely, because you've been able to knock out some of the answer choices that you know are wrong. If you are eliminating choices and realize that the last answer choice you are left with is also obviously wrong, don't panic. Start over and consider each choice again. There may easily be something that you missed the first time and will realize on the second pass.

Tough Questions

If you are stumped on a problem or it appears too hard or too difficult, don't waste time. Move on! Remember though, if you can quickly check for obviously incorrect answer choices, your chances of guessing correctly are greatly improved. Before you completely give up, at least try to knock out a couple of possible answers. Eliminate what you can and then guess at the remaining answer choices before moving on.

Brainstorm

If you get stuck on a difficult question, spend a few seconds quickly brainstorming. Run through the complete list of possible answer choices. Look at each choice and ask yourself, "Could this answer the question satisfactorily?" Go through each answer choice and consider it independently of the other. By systematically going through all possibilities, you may find something that you would otherwise overlook. Remember that when you get stuck, it's important to try to keep moving.

Read Carefully

Understand the problem. Read the question and answer choices carefully. Don't miss the question because you misread the terms. You have plenty of time to read each question thoroughly and make sure you understand what is being asked. Yet a happy medium must be attained, so don't waste too much time. You must read carefully, but efficiently.

Face Value

When in doubt, use common sense. Always accept the situation in the problem at face value. Don't read too much into it. These problems will not require you to make huge leaps of logic. The test writers aren't trying to throw you off with a cheap trick. If you have to go beyond creativity and make a leap of logic in order to have an answer choice answer the question, then you should look at the other answer choices. Don't overcomplicate the problem by creating theoretical relationships or explanations that will warp time or space. These are normal problems rooted in reality. It's just that the applicable relationship or explanation may not be readily apparent and you have to figure things out. Use your common sense to interpret anything that isn't clear.

Prefixes

If you're having trouble with a word in the question or answer choices, try dissecting it. Take advantage of every clue that the word might include. Prefixes and suffixes can be a huge help. Usually they allow you to determine a basic meaning. Pre- means before, post- means after, pro - is positive, de- is negative. From these prefixes and suffixes, you can get an idea of the general meaning of the word and try to put it into context. Beware though of any traps. Just because con is the opposite of pro, doesn't necessarily mean congress is the opposite of progress!

Hedge Phrases

Watch out for critical "hedge" phrases, such as likely, may, can, will often, sometimes, often, almost, mostly, usually, generally, rarely, sometimes. Question writers insert these hedge phrases to cover every possibility. Often an answer choice will be wrong simply because it leaves no room for exception. Avoid answer choices that have definitive words like "exactly," and "always".

Switchback Words

Stay alert for "switchbacks". These are the words and phrases frequently used to alert you to shifts in thought. The most common switchback word is "but". Others include although, however, nevertheless, on the other hand, even though, while, in spite of, despite, regardless of.

New Information

Correct answer choices will rarely have completely new information included. Answer choices typically are straightforward reflections of the material asked about and will directly relate to the question. If a new piece of information is included in an answer choice that doesn't even seem to relate to the topic being asked about, then that answer choice is likely incorrect. All of the information needed to answer the question is usually provided for you, and so you should not have to make guesses that are unsupported or choose answer choices that require unknown information that cannot be reasoned on its own.

Time Management

On technical questions, don't get lost on the technical terms. Don't spend too much time on any one question. If you don't know what a term means, then since you don't have a dictionary, odds are you aren't going to get much further. You should immediately recognize terms as whether or not you know them. If you don't, work with the other clues that you have, the other answer choices and terms provided, but don't waste too much time trying to figure out a difficult term.

Contextual Clues

Look for contextual clues. An answer can be right but not correct. The contextual clues will help you find the answer that is most right and is correct. Understand the context in which a phrase or statement is made. This will help you make important distinctions.

Don't Panic

Panicking will not answer any questions for you. Therefore, it isn't helpful. When you first see the question, if your mind goes blank, take a deep breath. Force yourself to mechanically go through the steps of solving the problem and using the strategies you've learned.

Pace Yourself

Don't get clock fever. It's easy to be overwhelmed when you're looking at a page full of questions, your mind is full of random thoughts and feeling confused, and the clock is ticking down faster than you would like. Calm down and maintain the pace that you have set for yourself. As long as you are on track by monitoring your pace, you are guaranteed to have enough time for yourself. When you get to the last few minutes of the test, it may seem like you won't have enough time left, but if you only have as many questions as you should have left at that point, then you're right on track!

Answer Selection

The best way to pick an answer choice is to eliminate all of those that are wrong, until only one is left and confirm that is the correct answer. Sometimes though, an answer choice may immediately look right. Be careful! Take a second to make sure that the other choices are not equally obvious. Don't make a hasty mistake. There are only two times that you should stop before checking other answers. First is when you are positive that the answer choice you have selected is correct. Second is when time is almost out and you have to make a quick guess!

Check Your Work

Since you will probably not know every term listed and the answer to every question, it is important that you get credit for the ones that you do know. Don't miss any questions through careless mistakes. If at all possible, try to take a second to look back over your answer selection and make sure you've selected the correct answer choice and haven't made a costly careless mistake (such as marking an answer choice that you didn't mean to mark). This quick double check should more than pay for itself in caught mistakes for the time it costs.

Beware of Directly Quoted Answers

Sometimes an answer choice will repeat word for word a portion of the question or reference section. However, beware of such exact duplication – it may be a trap! More than likely, the correct choice will paraphrase or summarize a point, rather than being exactly the same wording.

Slang

Scientific sounding answers are better than slang ones. An answer choice that begins "To compare the outcomes…" is much more likely to be correct than one that begins "Because some people insisted…"

Extreme Statements

Avoid wild answers that throw out highly controversial ideas that are proclaimed as established fact. An answer choice that states the "process should be used in certain situations, if…" is much more likely to be correct than one that states the "process should be discontinued completely." The first is a calm rational statement and doesn't even make a definitive, uncompromising stance, using a hedge word "if" to provide wiggle room, whereas the second choice is a radical idea and far more extreme.

Answer Choice Families

When you have two or more answer choices that are direct opposites or parallels, one of them is usually the correct answer. For instance, if one answer choice states "x increases" and another answer choice states "x decreases" or "y increases," then those two or three answer choices are very similar in construction and fall into the same family of answer choices. A family of answer choices is when two or three answer choices are very similar in construction, and yet often have a directly opposite meaning. Usually the correct answer choice will be in that family of answer choices. The "odd man out" or answer choice that doesn't seem to fit the parallel construction of the other answer choices is more likely to be incorrect.

Special Report: How to Overcome Test Anxiety

The very nature of tests caters to some level of anxiety, nervousness or tension, just as we feel for any important event that occurs in our lives. A little bit of anxiety or nervousness can be a good thing. It helps us with motivation, and makes achievement just that much sweeter. However, too much anxiety can be a problem; especially if it hinders our ability to function and perform.

"Test anxiety," is the term that refers to the emotional reactions that some test-takers experience when faced with a test or exam. Having a fear of testing and exams is based upon a rational fear, since the test-taker's performance can shape the course of an academic career. Nevertheless, experiencing excessive fear of examinations will only interfere with the test-takers ability to perform, and his/her chances to be successful.

There are a large variety of causes that can contribute to the development and sensation of test anxiety. These include, but are not limited to lack of performance and worrying about issues surrounding the test.

Lack of Preparation

Lack of preparation can be identified by the following behaviors or situations:

Not scheduling enough time to study, and therefore cramming the night before the test or exam
Managing time poorly, to create the sensation that there is not enough time to do everything
Failing to organize the text information in advance, so that the study material consists of the entire text and not simply the pertinent information
Poor overall studying habits

Worrying, on the other hand, can be related to both the test taker, or many other factors around him/her that will be affected by the results of the test. These include worrying about:

Previous performances on similar exams, or exams in general
How friends and other students are achieving
The negative consequences that will result from a poor grade or failure

There are three primary elements to test anxiety. Physical components, which involve the same typical bodily reactions as those to acute anxiety (to be discussed below). Emotional factors have to do with fear or panic. Mental or cognitive issues concerning attention spans and memory abilities.

Physical Signals

There are many different symptoms of test anxiety, and these are not limited to mental and emotional strain. Frequently there are a range of physical signals that will let a test taker know that he/she is suffering from test anxiety. These bodily changes can include the following:

Perspiring
Sweaty palms
Wet, trembling hands
Nausea
Dry mouth
A knot in the stomach
Headache
Faintness
Muscle tension
Aching shoulders, back and neck
Rapid heart beat
Feeling too hot/cold

To recognize the sensation of test anxiety, a test-taker should monitor him/herself for the following sensations:

The physical distress symptoms as listed above
Emotional sensitivity, expressing emotional feelings such as the need to cry or laugh too much, or a sensation of anger or helplessness
A decreased ability to think, causing the test-taker to blank out or have racing thoughts that are hard to organize or control.

Though most students will feel some level of anxiety when faced with a test or exam, the majority can cope with that anxiety and maintain it at a manageable level. However, those who cannot are faced with a very real and very serious condition, which can and should be controlled for the immeasurable benefit of this sufferer.

Naturally, these sensations lead to negative results for the testing experience. The most common effects of test anxiety have to do with nervousness and mental blocking.

Nervousness

Nervousness can appear in several different levels:

The test-taker's difficulty, or even inability to read and understand the questions on the test
The difficulty or inability to organize thoughts to a coherent form
The difficulty or inability to recall key words and concepts relating to the testing questions (especially essays)
The receipt of poor grades on a test, though the test material was well known by the test taker

Conversely, a person may also experience mental blocking, which involves:

Blanking out on test questions
Only remembering the correct answers to the questions when the test has already finished.

Fortunately for test anxiety sufferers, beating these feelings, to a large degree, has to do with proper preparation. When a test taker has a feeling of preparedness, then anxiety will be dramatically lessened.

The first step to resolving anxiety issues is to distinguish which of the two types of anxiety are being suffered. If the anxiety is a direct result of a lack of preparation, this should be considered a normal reaction, and the anxiety level (as opposed to the test results) shouldn't be anything to worry about. However, if, when adequately prepared, the test-taker still panics, blanks out, or seems to overreact, this is not a fully rational reaction. While this can be considered normal too, there are many ways to combat and overcome these effects.

Remember that anxiety cannot be entirely eliminated, however, there are ways to minimize it, to make the anxiety easier to manage. Preparation is one of the best ways to minimize test anxiety. Therefore the following techniques are wise in order to best fight off any anxiety that may want to build.

To begin with, try to avoid cramming before a test, whenever it is possible. By trying to memorize an entire term's worth of information in one day, you'll be shocking your system, and not giving yourself a very good chance to absorb the information. This is an easy path to anxiety, so for those who suffer from test anxiety, cramming should not even be considered an option.

Instead of cramming, work throughout the semester to combine all of the material which is presented throughout the semester, and work on it gradually as the course goes by, making sure to master the main concepts first, leaving minor details for a week or so before the test.

To study for the upcoming exam, be sure to pose questions that may be on the examination, to gauge the ability to answer them by integrating the ideas from your texts, notes and lectures, as well as any supplementary readings.

If it is truly impossible to cover all of the information that was covered in that particular term, concentrate on the most important portions, that can be covered very well. Learn these concepts as best as possible, so that when the test comes, a goal can be made to use these concepts as presentations of your knowledge.

In addition to study habits, changes in attitude are critical to beating a struggle with test anxiety. In fact, an improvement of the perspective over the entire test-taking experience can actually help a test taker to enjoy studying and therefore improve the overall experience. Be certain not to overemphasize the significance of the grade - know that the result of the test is neither a reflection of self worth, nor is it a measure of intelligence; one grade will not predict a person's future success.

To improve an overall testing outlook, the following steps should be tried:

Keeping in mind that the most reasonable expectation for taking a test is to expect to try to demonstrate as much of what you know as you possibly can. Reminding ourselves that a test is only one test; this is not the only one, and there will be others.
The thought of thinking of oneself in an irrational, all-or-nothing term should be avoided at all costs.
A reward should be designated for after the test, so there's something to look forward to. Whether it be going to a movie, going out to eat, or simply visiting friends, schedule it in advance, and do it no matter what result is expected on the exam.

Test-takers should also keep in mind that the basics are some of the most important things, even beyond anti-anxiety techniques and studying. Never neglect the basic social, emotional and biological needs, in order to try to absorb information. In order to best achieve, these three factors must be held as just as important as the studying itself.

Study Steps

Remember the following important steps for studying:

Maintain healthy nutrition and exercise habits. Continue both your recreational activities and social pass times. These both contribute to your physical and emotional well being.

Be certain to get a good amount of sleep, especially the night before the test, because when you're overtired you are not able to perform to the best of your best ability.

Keep the studying pace to a moderate level by taking breaks when they are needed, and varying the work whenever possible, to keep the mind fresh instead of getting bored.

When enough studying has been done that all the material that can be learned has been learned, and the test taker is prepared for the test, stop studying and do something relaxing such as listening to music, watching a movie, or taking a warm bubble bath.

There are also many other techniques to minimize the uneasiness or apprehension that is experienced along with test anxiety before, during, or even after the examination. In fact, there are a great deal of things that can be done to stop anxiety from interfering with lifestyle and performance. Again, remember that anxiety will not be eliminated entirely, and it shouldn't be. Otherwise that "up" feeling for exams would not exist, and most of us depend on that sensation to perform better than usual. However, this anxiety has to be at a level that is manageable.

Of course, as we have just discussed, being prepared for the exam is half the battle right away. Attending all classes, finding out what knowledge will be expected on the exam, and knowing the exam schedules are easy steps to lowering anxiety. Keeping up with work will remove the need to cram, and efficient study habits will eliminate wasted time. Studying should be done in an ideal location for concentration, so that it is simple to become interested in the material and give it complete attention. A method such as SQ3R (Survey, Question, Read, Recite, Review) is a wonderful key to follow to make sure that the study habits are as effective as possible, especially in the case of learning from a textbook. Flashcards are great techniques for memorization. Learning to take good notes will mean that notes will be full of useful information, so that less sifting will need to be done to seek out what is pertinent for studying. Reviewing notes after class and then again on occasion will keep the information fresh in the mind. From notes that have been taken summary sheets and outlines can be made for simpler reviewing.

A study group can also be a very motivational and helpful place to study, as there will be a sharing of ideas, all of the minds can work together, to make sure that everyone understands, and the studying will be made more interesting because it will be a social occasion.

Basically, though, as long as the test-taker remains organized and self confident, with efficient study habits, less time will need to be spent studying, and higher grades will be achieved.

To become self confident, there are many useful steps. The first of these is "self talk." It has been shown through extensive research, that self-talk for students who suffer from test anxiety, should be well monitored, in order to make sure that it contributes to self confidence as opposed to sinking the student. Frequently the self talk of test-anxious students is negative or self-defeating, thinking that everyone else is smarter and faster, that they always mess up, and that if they don't do well, they'll fail the entire course. It is important to decreasing anxiety that awareness is made of self talk. Try writing any negative self thoughts and then disputing them with a positive statement instead. Begin self-encouragement as though it was a friend speaking. Repeat positive statements to help reprogram the mind to believing in successes instead of failures.

Helpful Techniques

Other extremely helpful techniques include:

Self-visualization of doing well and reaching goals
While aiming for an "A" level of understanding, don't try to "overprotect" by setting your expectations lower. This will only convince the mind to stop studying in order to meet the lower expectations.
Don't make comparisons with the results or habits of other students. These are individual factors, and different things work for different people, causing different results.
Strive to become an expert in learning what works well, and what can be done in order to improve. Consider collecting this data in a journal.
Create rewards for after studying instead of doing things before studying that will only turn into avoidance behaviors.
Make a practice of relaxing - by using methods such as progressive relaxation, self-hypnosis, guided imagery, etc - in order to make relaxation an automatic sensation.
Work on creating a state of relaxed concentration so that concentrating will take on the focus of the mind, so that none will be wasted on worrying.
Take good care of the physical self by eating well and getting enough sleep.
Plan in time for exercise and stick to this plan.

Beyond these techniques, there are other methods to be used before, during and after the test that will help the test-taker perform well in addition to overcoming anxiety.

Before the exam comes the academic preparation. This involves establishing a study schedule and beginning at least one week before the actual date of the test. By doing this, the anxiety of not having enough time to study for the test will be automatically eliminated. Moreover, this will make the studying a much more effective experience, ensuring that the learning will be an easier process. This relieves much undue pressure on the test-taker.

Summary sheets, note cards, and flash cards with the main concepts and examples of these main concepts should be prepared in advance of the actual studying time. A topic should never be eliminated from this process. By omitting a topic because it isn't expected to be on the test is only setting up the test-taker for anxiety should it actually appear on the exam. Utilize the course syllabus for laying out the topics that should be studied. Carefully go over the notes that were made in class, paying special attention to any of the issues that the professor took special care to emphasize while lecturing in class. In the textbooks, use the chapter review, or if possible, the chapter tests, to begin your review.

It may even be possible to ask the instructor what information will be covered on the exam, or what the format of the exam will be (for example, multiple choice, essay, free form, true-false). Additionally, see if it is possible to find out how many questions will be on the test. If a review sheet or sample test has been offered by the professor, make good use of it, above anything else, for the preparation for the test. Another great resource for getting to know the examination is reviewing tests from previous semesters. Use these tests to review, and aim to achieve a 100% score on each of the possible topics. With a few exceptions, the goal that you set for yourself is the highest one that you will reach.

Take all of the questions that were assigned as homework, and rework them to any other possible course material. The more problems reworked, the more skill and confidence will form as a result. When forming the solution to a problem, write out each of the steps. Don't simply do head work. By doing as many steps on paper as possible, much clarification and therefore confidence will be formed. Do this with as many homework problems as possible, before checking the answers. By checking the answer after each problem, a reinforcement will exist, that will not be on the exam. Study situations should be as exam-like as possible, to prime the test-taker's system for the experience. By waiting to check the answers at the end, a psychological advantage will be formed, to decrease the stress factor.

Another fantastic reason for not cramming is the avoidance of confusion in concepts, especially when it comes to mathematics. 8-10 hours of study will become one hundred percent more effective if it is spread out over a week or at least several days, instead of doing it all in one sitting. Recognize that the human brain requires time in order to assimilate new material, so frequent breaks and a span of study time over several days will be much more beneficial.

Additionally, don't study right up until the point of the exam. Studying should stop a minimum of one hour before the exam begins. This allows the brain to rest and put things in their proper order. This will also provide the time to become as relaxed as possible when going into the examination room. The test-taker will also have time to eat well and eat sensibly. Know that the brain needs food as much as the rest of the body. With enough food and enough sleep, as well as a relaxed attitude, the body and the mind are primed for success.

Avoid any anxious classmates who are talking about the exam. These students only spread anxiety, and are not worth sharing the anxious sentimentalities.

Before the test also involves creating a positive attitude, so mental preparation should also be a point of concentration. There are many keys to creating a positive attitude. Should fears become rushing in, make a visualization of taking the exam, doing well, and seeing an A written on the paper. Write out a list of affirmations that will bring a feeling of confidence, such as "I am doing well in my English class," "I studied well and know my material," "I enjoy this class." Even if the affirmations aren't believed at first, it sends a positive message to the subconscious which will result in an alteration of the overall belief system, which is the system that creates reality.

If a sensation of panic begins, work with the fear and imagine the very worst! Work through the entire scenario of not passing the test, failing the entire course, and dropping out of school, followed by not getting a job, and pushing a shopping cart through the dark alley where you'll live. This will place things into perspective! Then, practice deep breathing and create a visualization of the opposite situation - achieving an "A" on the exam, passing the entire course, receiving the degree at a graduation ceremony.

On the day of the test, there are many things to be done to ensure the best results, as well as the most calm outlook. The following stages are suggested in order to maximize test-taking potential:

Begin the examination day with a moderate breakfast, and avoid any coffee or beverages with caffeine if the test taker is prone to jitters. Even people who are used to managing caffeine can feel jittery or light-headed when it is taken on a test day.
Attempt to do something that is relaxing before the examination begins. As last minute cramming clouds the mastering of overall concepts, it is better to use this time to create a calming outlook.

Be certain to arrive at the test location well in advance, in order to provide time to select a location that is away from doors, windows and other distractions, as well as giving enough time to relax before the test begins.

Keep away from anxiety generating classmates who will upset the sensation of stability and relaxation that is being attempted before the exam.

Should the waiting period before the exam begins cause anxiety, create a self-distraction by reading a light magazine or something else that is relaxing and simple.

During the exam itself, read the entire exam from beginning to end, and find out how much time should be allotted to each individual problem. Once writing the exam, should more time be taken for a problem, it should be abandoned, in order to begin another problem. If there is time at the end, the unfinished problem can always be returned to and completed.

Read the instructions very carefully - twice - so that unpleasant surprises won't follow during or after the exam has ended.

When writing the exam, pretend that the situation is actually simply the completion of homework within a library, or at home. This will assist in forming a relaxed atmosphere, and will allow the brain extra focus for the complex thinking function.

Begin the exam with all of the questions with which the most confidence is felt. This will build the confidence level regarding the entire exam and will begin a quality momentum. This will also create encouragement for trying the problems where uncertainty resides.

Going with the "gut instinct" is always the way to go when solving a problem. Second guessing should be avoided at all costs. Have confidence in the ability to do well.

For essay questions, create an outline in advance that will keep the mind organized and make certain that all of the points are remembered. For multiple choice, read every answer, even if the correct one has been spotted - a better one may exist.

Continue at a pace that is reasonable and not rushed, in order to be able to work carefully. Provide enough time to go over the answers at the end, to check for small errors that can be corrected.

Should a feeling of panic begin, breathe deeply, and think of the feeling of the body releasing sand through its pores. Visualize a calm, peaceful place, and include all of the sights, sounds and sensations of this image. Continue the deep breathing, and take a few minutes to continue this with closed eyes. When all is well again, return to the test.

If a "blanking" occurs for a certain question, skip it and move on to the next question. There will be time to return to the other question later. Get everything done that can be done, first, to guarantee all the grades that can be compiled, and to build all of the confidence possible. Then return to the weaker questions to build the marks from there.

Remember, one's own reality can be created, so as long as the belief is there, success will follow. And remember: anxiety can happen later, right now, there's an exam to be written!

After the examination is complete, whether there is a feeling for a good grade or a bad grade, don't dwell on the exam, and be certain to follow through on the reward that was promised…and enjoy it! Don't dwell on any mistakes that have been made, as there is nothing that can be done at this point anyway.

Additionally, don't begin to study for the next test right away. Do something relaxing for a while, and let the mind relax and prepare itself to begin absorbing information again.

From the results of the exam - both the grade and the entire experience, be certain to learn from what has gone on. Perfect studying habits and work some more on confidence in order to make the next examination experience even better than the last one.

Learn to avoid places where openings occurred for laziness, procrastination and day dreaming.

Use the time between this exam and the next one to better learn to relax, even learning to relax on cue, so that any anxiety can be controlled during the next exam. Learn how to relax the body. Slouch in your chair if that helps. Tighten and then relax all of the different muscle groups, one group at a time, beginning with the feet and then working all the way up to the neck and face. This will ultimately relax the muscles more than they were to begin with. Learn how to breathe deeply and comfortably, and focus on this breathing going in and out as a relaxing thought. With every exhale, repeat the word "relax."

As common as test anxiety is, it is very possible to overcome it. Make yourself one of the test-takers who overcome this frustrating hindrance.

Special Report: Additional Bonus Material

Due to our efforts to try to keep this book to a manageable length, we've created a link that will give you access to all of your additional bonus material.

Please visit http://www.mometrix.com/bonus948/certmedasst to access the information.